T0285275

want

want

Submitted by anonymous

Collected by
gillian anderson

ABRAMS PRESS | NEW YORK

Library of Congress Control Number: 2024935810

ISBN: 978-1-4197-7729-5
eISBN: 979-8-88707-433-7

Printed and bound in the United States
10 9 8 7 6 5 4 3 2 1

ABRAMS The Art of Books
195 Broadway, New York, NY 10007
abramsbooks.com

contents

key

We asked every contributor certain facts about themselves and we've included their answers at the end of each letter. Some contributors didn't answer every question and in those situations it says NA.

Ethnic group and nationality
Religion
Annual income
Sexual orientation
Relationship status
Children

introduction

I was barely *five years old in 1973 when the novelist Nancy Friday's cult classic*, My Secret Garden: Women's Sexual Fantasies, *made its way onto the bookshelves and into the handbags of women in the US; just seven when it reached the women of Middle England.* My Secret Garden *was proof that women enjoyed as rich and diverse an erotic inner life as men. Finally, here was a book in which ordinary women, young and old – 'you, me and our next-door neighbour' – were talking honestly about arousal, masturbation, sexual dreams and desires. In their minds, nothing was off limits.*

What Friday's book revealed was that, for some of us, the sex we have in our head may be more stimulating than the physical nuts and bolts of any coupling, no matter how hot. Unconstrained by assumed social conventions, self-consciousness or perhaps the fear of making our partners uncomfortable, in our imaginations we can indulge in our deepest, most transgressive desires. It was provocative, even revolutionary, at the start, and then it became required reading, a multimillion-copy global bestseller.

I don't know if my computer analyst mother owned a copy of Friday's book. Ours certainly wasn't a puritanical household where such reading matter would have been frowned upon – but as liberal as my childhood was, it wouldn't have been something that Mom left lying about on the coffee table. When I was a teenager, I once found a copy of Story of O, *the infamous French erotic novel by Anne Desclos, tucked behind a sofa cushion in our neighbours' house and I definitely turned a few pages. And as a much younger child, I remember wandering into a living room where someone had left the TV on, and standing paralysed in fascination as the on-screen couple engaged in quite chaste but clearly illicit activities. I can still recall my red-hot cheeks, quickened heartbeat and palpable rising shame.*

I read My Secret Garden *for the first time when I was preparing for my role as the sex therapist Dr Jean Milburn in the TV series* Sex Education. *The letters and interviews were astonishingly intimate and very raw. Their unfiltered and painful honesty shook me. They weren't polished, or trying to be literary; they seemed to come straight from the mysterious heart of women's innermost yearning. The human imagination has few limits and our sexual desires and fantasies are no different, yet are still treated as taboo. Friday conceived the book as a response to a male editor's objection to an erotic fantasy in one of her novels, a response considered so dangerous it was banned in the Republic of Ireland. Bringing female fantasies into the open also brought up contentious questions – did women want to act on these imaginings? What did it mean to have a fantasy that was unusual, forbidden or even illegal? What might it tell us about the established gender roles that had been foisted upon women?*

So much has changed in our social and sexual relations in the fifty years since My Secret Garden *was first published. Have women's deepest internal desires also changed? I am a woman, with a sex life and fantasies of my own, and I was curious to know the ways in which a diverse group of other women's fantasies were similar to, or different from, mine.*

The book you hold in your hands started as an invitation to women across the globe. 'Dear Gillian' was a call for women to share the sexual fantasies, thoughts and feelings that so many of us hold in our heads but so rarely speak out loud. A chance to gather the voices of women worldwide into a new book of fantasies for a new generation. My publishers set up a portal where the letters could be sent anonymously. And we waited … We had so many questions: might women find something interesting or erotic in putting pen to paper and sharing their inner thoughts with others? Indeed, what would change as we made the intrinsically private public? How would people respond? At the close of the submission deadline, the combined letters counted 800,000 words – we had received enough entries to fill at least eight volumes. Clearly, there was a need.

The call for letters unleashed a torrent of frank, candid, heart-breaking, funny and downright raunchy outpourings which highlighted fantasies as rich and varied as the authors themselves. Letters from women who had never articulated – either out loud or on paper – their sexual secrets to anyone before, save for the odd morsel they let slip over drinks with a close friend or in the heat of the moment with a partner. It was obvious that participating in 'Dear Gillian' was, for them, a process that felt both liberating and illicit. There were letters from teenage girls yet to have their first sexual encounter; from single women caught in the endless cycle of online hook-ups and one-night stands; exhausted women with young children; married women or those with long-term partners frustrated with the same old, same old; transgender women and people who identify as non-binary; and women in their sixties and seventies, finding that there's much to shout about in post-menopausal sex. Here were letters from women all over the world – from Colombia to China, Ireland to Iceland, Lithuania to Libya, New Zealand to Nigeria, Romania to Russia. Letters from women who are pansexual, bisexual, asexual, aromantic, lesbian, straight and queer.

As a society, we habitually put women into boxes, limiting and constraining their identities and roles – the enticing sexual partner, the caring mother, the smart career woman – and yet what these fantasies demonstrate is that no woman has one sole identity. I wanted to challenge the categorisations that women are forced into; and yet! A book must have structure and order! It made the process of putting the book together both challenging and fascinating: I found *huge pleasure in the process of juxtaposing the letters, creating a system and watching it take shape in a kind of rhythm that at times felt poetic. The submissions have also made me consider my own identity: the labels of actor, mother, partner, activist, American/ British woman. And so, with this in mind and in the spirit of this project, I too submitted my own letter to the book. I was curious to see how it fitted in; would it blend in naturally, and would it match people's assumptions about me (though we will never know)?*

For me, sex has never felt like a static entity but rather something that adapts and changes as I grow and change, with every new phase and stage of my life. A huge part of this has always been in the thinking and the feeling, not just the doing. As an actor, there is an inherent permission at the core of my job to give myself over to an alternate reality, which is the very definition of fantasy. The women whom I embody, whose worlds I step into, also have inner lives, desires and fantasies, which are vital to understanding what makes them tick. And a fair few of them have taught me about sex and sexuality.

When I first read My Secret Garden, *what struck me most was women's overriding sense of shame. For women in 1973, admitting their inner sexual desires to themselves, never mind other people, was fraught with internal discomfort. Surely, I thought, things would be different in the twenty-first century? What with greater visibility of LGBTQIA+ communities, the multibillion-dollar porn industry, and TV drama series like* Sex Education, Euphoria *and* Normal People *attracting viewers in the tens of millions, these must be thoughts and conversations women have all the time? Well, not entirely.*

I found it surprising that a great number of women today continue to keep their fantasies to themselves. Many of those who wrote to me are loud, proud, confident women owning and celebrating their sexual power, but just as many expressed feeling shame and guilt in seeking sexual comfort and satisfaction. As one contributor writes,

'I often find myself questioning the shame that comes along with my desires. Is everyone ashamed and pretending not to be?' There are plenty for whom sexual fantasies can only ever be secret. It was sobering to read the first-hand experience of those living in countries where social norms – or, in some cases, the law – precludes the possibility of anything other than a heterosexual relationship and sex within marriage. But even contributors from so-called liberal societies write of feeling 'shame', 'embarrassment' or 'guilt', of their fear or reluctance to talk to a partner about what they truly think about when they are having sex with them or, often, when masturbating alone.

But, and this is a very big but: I am not an expert and have no professional qualifications in this area. I am an actor by trade, and will therefore not be analysing these letters, or offering explanations on womanhood or sex in general. What I can do, though, dear reader, is present them to you, so that you may savour these extraordinary letters without a filter. I have always been intrigued by sexual fantasies and I view my role in this book as that of a curator, shepherding these diverse and amazing voices into book form. It has been an incredible journey and so gratifying to see how different we all are but also how much we are the same the world over. This book is a platform for the voices of women, to enable us, in complete anonymity, not only to share but, paradoxically, to be seen and heard. I want to remove the taboo of fantasies and bring in the thrill and the fun in the hope that this book, these letters, through disclosure, representation and identification, might inspire.

Reading the letters gave me so much more than simply an insight into women's imaginary sexual worlds; it also granted me a look-in to the circumstances in which fantasies come into play. For many women, fantasies fulfil a vital role as a means of escape, a retreat from the pressures and demands of work and parenthood, the mundanity of everyday life. As one contributor explains, sexual fantasies have long provided solace in a lonely marriage: 'I would have sex twice a day if I could and he could happily live without it. He often made me feel ashamed for wanting sex, for wanting it too much and for expressing any desires. My fantasies became my companions from then on. Many of them would have themes of being totally free, spontaneous and wild.' It is perhaps unnerving that this letter sounds like it could have been written fifty years ago to Nancy Friday – in some parts of women's lives, nothing has changed. For some women, sexual fantasies can be a lifeline. As one letter reads, 'I feel like fantasising gives me the will to live.' For others, fantasies are a prompt to enhance their arousal and are an addition, not a replacement, for an adventurous sex life.

The potent thing about all intentional sexual fantasies is that we are the authors of the stories. We have agency and we control the action, who does what to whom and how, down to the last elaborate, exquisite, erotic detail. We can choose to do whatever we want, with whomever we want, however many people we want, whenever we want – without fear, without societal judgement or consequence. I think that's key: fantasy can help crystallise our wants and needs. It can free us to explore ourselves, to experiment with our arousal and our desire without risk of harm or criticism. Fantasy is a safe space; it is not necessarily what we wish was real. Crucially, in a fantasy we don't need anyone's permission other than our own: a fantasy is a deliberate, and usually entirely private, act of both memory and imagination.

Indeed, sometimes, where reality fails, fantasy comes into play. In many letters, the author's satisfaction and arousal is linked to how sexy they feel or how they worry about being perceived. Some women write that they are unable to include their real selves in their own fantasies – they imagine they are the man at the centre of the action, or an unknown woman, or some flawless version of themselves, 'younger and with perkier breasts'. These idealised sexual fantasies are clearly a safe means of escape from self-judgement, self-consciousness, body and performance insecurity. We can let ourselves go, be our best, sexiest, hottest selves, and stop worrying about the 'perfect' body, postpartum weight or having varicose veins. As this woman says: 'I have a very difficult time navigating what really turns me on vs how I feel I should perform. I guess my number one fantasy is to be made to feel like I am utterly desired. Not because it's just another naked body, but because it's me and my body.'

So, what do we fantasise about, and why? Well, as you will see, the sexual fantasies we received are as richly diverse as the women who wrote them. The widespread influence of erotic fiction, such as E. L. James's Fifty Shades of Grey (2011), on your deepest desires is loud and clear and another differentiating factor from My Secret Garden, demonstrating signs of a society more familiar with a wider erotic vocabulary. There are fantasies of BDSM between consenting adults in both the dominant and submissive roles, and others relating to the switch between them. Fantasies featuring rope play and spanking, paddles and whips, blindfolds and handcuffs, choking and restraint, anal plugs, dildos and vibrators of every shape and size. Interestingly, many of the letters that detail dreams of being dominated and ceding control come from women who describe careers that come with great responsibility and power, as well as being largely responsible for keeping the house and family life on track. I also found fascinating that some women fantasise about being a 'hucow', a new term for me (essentially, being milked). Many more described fantasies of having unprotected sex and of wanting to experience the sensation of a man coming inside them. This certainly marks a generational divide — for the post-AIDS generation, protected sex is the norm. These successive generations have also come of age in the throes of the technological and digital revolution, which has evidently manifested in our erotic lives, and not solely in the form of 24/7 access to porn. Several women see the appeal of a fully functioning, highly realistic male robot that can satisfy their every *sexual whim — what was once the stuff of science fiction feels much less fantastical today.*

Yet many archetypal fantasies persist in their popularity. Included here are a mere fraction of the imagined threesomes and moresomes that we received, which current research shows are by far the most common sexual fantasies. Similarly, there were any number of fantasies about office sex with a colleague or boss; the risky kind of sex where someone might catch you in flagrante; voyeuristic sex, either as the participant or the observer; sex in front of an audience; sex with strangers; sex outdoors. More unexpected, perhaps, were the fantasies about sex with a tentacled alien or a half-human half-beast — suffice to say, we were spoilt for choice.

On a darker note, while we were anxious not to include letters that might trigger traumatic responses, it would be disingenuous not to acknowledge that some women do fantasise about being 'used' for sex, or about being abducted and raped by their kidnappers. But it is important to emphasise that these are fantasies. *And perhaps the purpose of fantasy is this: to provide a space where we can safely imagine and play out potentially dangerous and demeaning situations within the confines of our minds and our bedrooms.*

I was terrified of putting my own fantasy down on paper, lest someone was able to discern which was mine (let alone my publishers knowing more about me than I would necessarily wish them to!). If I'm honest, I think there are two sides to me, as perhaps there are to many women: the side that is good at asking for what I want and the side that will concede to my partner's desires, that is happy to share my innermost urges but only if my partner starts the conversation (and then not all of them). Is that due to shame? Or an indication that I wouldn't trust anyone with that level of intimacy? Or is it that I think it's somehow better to be, in part, unknowable? Do we all, in some way, struggle with being totally knowable?

As a sex and relationship therapist, Dr Jean Milburn, my character on Sex Education, would no doubt argue, it's incredibly healthy to share your innermost fantasies with your partner. She might say that this divulgence creates closeness, stimulates arousal and exhibits a level of trust that can only be beneficial to a sexual partnership. But then Jean has a fair few boundary issues of her own and I wouldn't trust her entirely on intimate relationships – doctorate or not. That is the world of television, and her dubious moral compass makes for great entertainment!

Nevertheless, even in the real world, from the moment the first series dropped on Netflix, it was evident that there was a vast audience ready for the show's frankness about all things sex. It isn't unusual for any of the characters, even the teenage ones, to speak openly about their deepest and darkest fantasies, and I'd wager a good number would be darker than most that are revealed in the pages of this book. The volume of submissions we received, however, and the degree of intimate detail divulged clearly indicate that many women want to share, they want to be heard, seen and validated – and, well, quite simply, they want. And so, our title.

I was also delighted to read just how many of the women ended their letters by noting the pleasure and sexual arousal they had experienced in the act of writing down their fantasies. You have no idea how much joy it gives me to imagine all of you beautiful women across the world, sitting down at your devices and typing away, articulating your sexual dreams, and pouring your deepest wants, desires and secrets onto the page. I am thrilled that so many of you are embracing your eroticism and, in the process, having a bloody good time.

Finally, a word on the selection and editing process. I want to thank everyone who took the time to write a letter to me. I have carefully read and considered every single one. Unfortunately, much as I would have loved to include every letter, a 1,000-page book was just not a feasible option. I apologise if your letter has not been included – this is not a reflection on either the fantasy you described or the quality of your writing. My aim was to gather as wide a range of voices as possible, from different nations, sexual identities, religions and backgrounds. When we asked for demographic details from our contributors, we asked about sexual identity, but not gender identity. Though an imperfect term, 'women' is used throughout. This speaks to the gendered way we understand fantasies; the contributors in this book, both women and genderqueer people, know what it means to have their voices and wants downplayed within a patriarchal society, where the fantasies of men take centre stage. The wider our spread of voices, the more we can really understand how women and genderqueer people feel about their sex lives today. Our first chapter is, fittingly, 'On Fantasies' – an introduction to this brilliant and varied selection of women's voices.

This project delivered so much more than I, or anyone involved, could have hoped for – a torrent of unbridled passion from across the world. I have been awed by the openness, self-awareness and natural eloquence with which you have expressed yourselves and the trust you've put in me to collate the responses. And if I have one hope for this book, it is that it will start a new conversation about sexual power, particularly for women. Sexual liberation must mean freedom to enjoy sex on our terms, to say what we want, not what we are pressured or believe we are expected to want. One thing is for sure: sexual fantasy continues to play a vital and healthy role in our lives as women and genderqueer people. And all of us have the power to say – and get – what we really, really WANT.

Gillian Anderson, April 2024

on fantasies

'I'll keep your secret if you keep mine.'
'*My* fantasies, my rules, right?'

I would like to understand myself. Not as a person, but as a human. I often find myself questioning the shame that comes along with my desires. Is everyone ashamed and pretending not to be? As humans – as animals – we are desiring individuals, and yet we think of ourselves as something bigger, more important than mammals: intelligent beings who founded cities and discovered how to use fire to cook vegetables, celebrating the result of organised sowed seeds.

I'm searching for answers. As a teenager, I lived as a lesbian, but what do I want now? I'm terrified of change: it's easier to label myself and stay trapped, but I'm sure I'd be a pretty sad woman. I want to touch and be touched, to love and be loved. I can't think of sex as an act lacking affection. I want someone to stroke my hair and my skin, someone to tell me that they desire me. I want to be worshipped and to worship, I care about the mutual act of making love. And at the same time, there's a part of me that wants to know how it feels to be fucked. Is it possible to be simultaneously attracted to cuteness *and* to roughness? To have a deep, primal desire of being controlled. It's the unknown, I think, that excites me.

As women, we do everything we can to be independent individuals. Immersed in a system that will do anything to make us the weaker gender, I find my desire in conflict with my rational thinking. Is this the reason I feel shame any time I think about being dominated? As much as we think of ourselves as powerful, we females are trained to feel shame from the day we are born. I, like many other women, feel shame about my body. And that's where the roots of my insecurities are: am I desirable in the way I look? I don't want to be objectified and yet I want to be desired. Maybe I'm just attracted to contradiction.

I want a relationship but I'm scared. And somehow my fears all add up to sex. I want someone to touch me, to fill me, to make me want to be touched. I want someone to tell me what to do and what to say, how to please them and when to stop. I want to be edged, to play with the limits. I want to trust someone to the point where I feel safe while being controlled. I want to moan from pleasure and also from pain. To be thrown over and to be fucked – even if it's a vague, common fantasy, it's not easy for me to assume the truth: I desire. My fantasies are limited by my rational self – which is embarrassed by *me*. I know that for sure. I'd like to let my mind run wild, but it is so, so hard.

I'll try, for you but especially for me: I finally learned that I like to dance, so I'm at a party, having a good time. I see someone I like but I'm not sure if they've noticed me, so I keep dancing. After a while, I feel a hand gently touching my back, so I turn round. When I see their face, I smile and dance along, feeling the increasing tension running through my skin. Slowly, as if previously planned, their hands go to my waist and mine go to their neck, their soft hair. Can't imagine how, but we're already kissing. It is a slow kiss, and my torso is closer to theirs as the minutes pass by. When the hands over my body start to make me feel like I need more, I suggest we go somewhere more private. We find a bathroom where we continue with the making out, with the touching. And as the hands go down, the adrenaline goes up, and the fact that we could be caught makes me more excited. They push me up against the cold, hard wall, with my face towards it. From the back, they put a hand under my long skirt and start to touch me over my underwear. The rubbing of the clothing against my clitoris turns me on, and when it starts to feel like I could come, they stop. And I ask them not to, but they shush me and tell me to turn and face them. As I do that, their hand goes up and to my mouth, where a finger meets my lips and then enters. I like my own flavour, it's a reminder of being alive. Then, as one hand is entering my mouth and playing with my tongue, the other one goes down and starts to rub my inner thighs, making me want more, so I ask for it. They don't do that.

Instead, they keep touching everything but the clitoris, and I'm so vulnerable standing there, waiting to be fucked and knowing that anyone could come through the door at any moment. When the hand goes to my clitoris my underwear is by my knees, so this time it is skin-to-skin. It's not the fingers but the entire hand that strokes me. I'm sensitive and it burns but just a little, the right amount to make me feel like I'm going to succumb. We are kissing but I need to take a deep breath, so I stop to catch some air. As I feel the need of being filled, they fill me. It's like they could read my thoughts, the desire of feeling them inside of me. Two fingers going inside and out, going slow but rough. I feel the music vibrating in my chest, the bass caressing my brain as I feel the sex as something that happens to me. Music and dancing, the lovemaking ritual.

Part of the fantasy is not knowing if I come, not caring if I do. In my mind I feel pleasure. Will I feel it in my body someday? To be touched, to be loved. To be a woman in love with the world she created.

[Argentine • <$19,000 • Gay/lesbian • Single • No]

I would like to have a penis. That is my fantasy. I love my boobs and my femininity. But I would like to have a penis to fuck a woman, or many women, with care and protection, but also with fiery desire and to feel the pleasure that men feel when having sex with a woman. And mostly to share the desire at the same time. That must feel amazing. Not so long ago I wished to be a man, or so I thought, because what I *really* wanted was to have the privileges that men have. Not only their rights and safety but, mostly, their penis.

I long for technology able to make me feel like I have a penis and give as much arousal and desire as possible to a woman. A hot, sexy, funny, lovely woman. 'Please send me one,' I asked the space that surrounds me, to my ideas, to you, I guess. Isn't that funny? I'm a bit desperate, but I try not to think too much about it. I guess for now I'll have to get a rubber penis and find a woman who wants to kiss me and have sex with me, to begin with. A hard task. I don't know whom to ask for advice or to introduce me to hot, funny, feminine women. And it sucks. I also don't think I am ugly at all, so I don't understand why I can't find a woman who would like to be with me. I don't think I have ever been loved by a woman, or by any romantic interest, as a matter of fact. It hurts. Sometimes my heart aches because of that silent rejection. Somehow, I feel lonely thinking about the fact that I can't find a female match on Tinder or Bumble, or in real life. It used to be easy on apps, for me. But now, it doesn't work. I sometimes feel I am in the wrong place and maybe also the wrong time.

And so, I want to escape to a foreign land, and I fantasise about the possibility of finding someone there who cherishes me and desires me. And loves me. I would like to experience that. Something healthy, something lovely, something comforting. And I don't just want sex. I want a sweet, real and honest connection, even if it is only for a while. For a tiny fraction of time. A sweet balm. I still want a penis, but I guess my biggest fantasy is to find someone to love. To really love and to be loved. Thank you for this space. Writing this has made me feel better.

[Mestiza Ecuadorean • <$19,000 • Bisexual/pansexual • Single • No]

As far as sex goes, fantasising is all I've ever done. I held hands with someone once a long time ago but that's it. I've always had an active fantasy life but the recent realisation that I'm not straight has amped things up. If people knew what I was thinking when I'm sitting at the kitchen table eating a cheese sandwich! Well, let's just say I could be imagining something completely different in my mouth.

It's confusing how much my fantasies have changed over the last couple of years. Before it was just two people in the missionary position, which is cool. You can still have a lot of fun that way, but now it's 'yes, please', to things that I wouldn't have dreamt of dreaming about before: BDSM (bondage, discipline, sadism, masochism), kink, three-or-moresomes, escorts, sex parties and clubs, watching and being watched, one-night hook-ups with random strangers. Anal sex and things I didn't even know were things until a year ago, like fisting. A current favourite fantasy is one where I'm at a party surrounded by people in various stages of undress, all engaged in different activities. My mouth is on someone's nipple, my hand is inside them and they're riding it and riding it until ...

Discovering my queerness has completely changed my thoughts and feelings about *everything*, not just sex and fantasies. It's like I've had a personality transplant. I mean, watching porn was a no-go area before, but now – women together, men together, men and women, groups, solo masturbation – I love it! I tend not to fantasise about real people (unless it's that delivery person with the tattoos and the undercut!). I do have inappropriate thoughts about people, though. You know, when you're talking to someone, and a thought just pops into your head? What do you taste like? What do you like doing in bed? What would your penis feel like in my hand right now? But mainly, it's just people I've made up in my imagination. The same person can be part of a long-term relationship, someone

8

I'm madly in love with, or a ten-minute encounter in a nightclub restroom. I do have special people that stay in my fantasies for a while but mainly it's *a lot* of different people. And before, I always dreamt about fit, good-looking, able-bodied people, but now it's every kind of person, every kind of body. Looks, gender, race and sexuality don't come into it. Age doesn't come into it either. My imaginary friends can be twenty-five or eighty-five and everything in between. But whatever kind of situation I find my imaginary self in, it's always unofficial. It seems I'm scared to even fantasise about full-time, out-and-proud relationships. That, however, doesn't stop me obsessing about throuples and polycules. When I heard about a possible celebrity throuple a few weeks ago, I broke out in a cold sweat and that day's fantasies were sorted.

I love how freewheeling fantasies can be. A chaste, loving relationship with someone asexual lives quite happily alongside several people I don't know very well giving it to me hard up against a wall. One minute, I could be walking down the street holding hands with someone, being all lovey-dovey; the next, I'm with several others in a dungeon, all of us dressed for the occasion, some strapped to a frame being punished, others wielding our whips with relish. Then there are times in my fantasy life when I'm travelling around the world, a sort of sexual nomad. I'm not interested in the sights of the foreign country, but seek out places, retreats, communes, clubs where I can meet like-minded people and have sex in as many ways as possible.

But I also kind of hate how free and easy fantasy can be. I mean, the whole point of fantasising is to make you feel good and it does sometimes; other times, though, I feel paralysed by it. I've just read a magazine article about someone falling in love with a woman for the first time. Instead of doing stuff that needed doing, I sat there staring at the page for ages imagining that it was happening to me. And it's pointless for me to try to watch television or read a book because I just can't focus on anything. I think I need therapy.

I thought that getting some of it out of my head and onto paper would help but writing it down like this has made me feel worse. It's made me see how selfish and indulgent I'm being. I'm sitting there watching the news with the latest tragedy playing out in front of me and my own life is a complete mess and the people around me need help, but all I can think about is bodies and fucking and relationships. It makes me feel ashamed. I know fantasies are supposed to be a distraction from real life, but it can be a burden. I dread waking up sometimes because I know it will all start before I even open my eyes. It feels like my life is made up of sex dreams punctuated by an occasional real-life event. It's also highlighted how frustrated I am. I wonder how different my fantasies would be if I was out there dating. Reading over what I've written, I think it might all be a bit naive and basic compared to what some other people fantasise about but ... *my* fantasies, my rules, right?

[Mixed-race British • <$19,000 • Bisexual/pansexual • Single • No]

I'm happily married. I think. My husband is a great guy. He's kind. He's easy to get on with. We have common interests. He's a great dad. He respects me. He works hard. He supports me financially. He's my best friend. And being married to your best friend is the best thing in the world. But sometimes I wonder how my life would be if he died. I wonder if I'd be brave. If my tastes would change. If I would be different from the twenty-year-old who fancied a guy who turned out to be her best friend and husband. If I'd be courageous enough to admit to myself, my family, my friends, my children, what I actually wanted.

I worked with a girl. I say girl, she was a woman. She was nothing like anyone I knew; long dark shiny hair, a huge smile, her teeth too big for her mouth, her arms covered in tattoos, small breasts. Her eyes glittered as they caught mine and saw past the tired bags, the shapeless cardigan hiding my baby belly. Her face was animated when I spoke; her body angled towards me. She was leaving to go abroad the next day. A few of us decided to have a drink. I remember exactly where I was when she came up behind me, her demeanour casual as she put her arm round my waist, her fingers entwining with mine. I refused to look down; instead stared ahead. I felt drunk. Felt my cheeks redden. My whole body was on fire as I stood there pretending to follow the conversation, smiling and nodding when I could. I inched backwards, my body skimming off hers; her face laughing at something someone had said. I smiled though I hadn't followed a word of the conversation. I shut my eyes for just a second, and then her hand dropped. The absence burned. And I stumbled sideways. I made my excuses and went home to my kids and my best friend. Now I see her only on Instagram. Or when I look in the bathroom mirror. I see her standing behind me. I see her holding my vibrator and I imagine my husband is dead. And I wonder if I'd be brave enough to let her work her way round my body. If I'd let her long hair tickle my breasts, if her petite chest would fit into my voluptuous one. Would I be brave enough to kiss her? Would I be bold enough to let her explore my body as I in turn explored hers? Would I be brave enough to share her with my children? I'm not brave enough now. I'm not brave enough to leave my husband. I'll never leave him. He's my best friend. We hold hands walking down the street, but in bed we face apart. Not from anger, but from tiredness. From contentment. Resignation. I'm resigned to a life of contentment. A happy life. No desires. Just conformity. Maybe being married to your best friend isn't all that bad.

[White British • Jewish • <$38,000 • Straight • Married/in a civil partnership • Yes]

I have a secret that I have never told anyone – if you pass me on the street, sitting on the metro, shopping in the supermarket, it's highly likely that I will be creating a detailed, smoking-hot sexual fantasy in my head. You might think I'm validating my travel pass, waiting for a green light at the pedestrian crossing or choosing fruit and veg, but in my head, I'm being taken from behind in the shower by a man whose name I don't even know. Or perhaps I'm flirting with a stranger in a bar, candlelight reflecting in my eyes and all sorts of promise for the evening ahead.

I live a perfectly fulfilling life – a job I enjoy, good friends, an active social life and a partner whom I love. But when I'm alone, engaged in the thousand and one mundanities of everyday life, that's when my elaborate alternative life begins. Sometimes these men (and the occasional woman) are famous figures – during a trip around the supermarket, I enjoy an extended daydream about a British rocker. After meeting in a bar, we end up in his cosy apartment with beautiful built-in bookcases jammed with records and books (it's not just the sex that is elaborately imagined) – and we begin to kiss. I taste the red wine we've been drinking and we move to the sofa. As things heat up, I slide onto his cock and he holds my hips, rocking me back and forth and whispering to me. As we climax, I pay for my items at the self-service checkout and leave. I see a handsome, serious politician giving a press conference and immediately imagine him in my apartment. He has brought me a gift – lingerie, black, lacy shorts-style knickers. I put them on and he kneels in front of me, gently pushes the underwear to one side and begins to caress me with his tongue. I come hard, gripping his thick dark hair with its peppering of grey. But more often these men are entirely imaginary. Thinking of some building work that I need to get done leads me to a classic, old-school porn fantasy of the bored housewife and the sexy builder. There was a strike that day so I had to walk all the way to work and our encounter lasted me for the entire hour-long duration of my journey.

I remember when I first discovered the thrill of an imaginary encounter while keeping a perfectly straight face in a public setting. My then boyfriend lent me a Prince CD and his Discman (yes, I'm that old) and I sat on the bus listening to his 'Orgasm' song, which, they said, featured a recording of a real sexual encounter. Who knows? These days I like to walk around my city, which is unusually picturesque, sometimes listening to music and often weaving my fantasies as I go – and then for the rest of the day I interact with the world in a perfectly normal fashion. So next time you see an entirely unremarkable woman walking down the street, wearing a slight smile – she might be me.

[White British • <$64,000 • Heterosexual • In a relationship • No]

I've found it so difficult to understand what, truly, my own fantasies are. So much of what is played out in porn is geared towards men, and so many expectations set on us as women, that I have a very difficult time navigating what really turns me on vs how I feel I *should* perform. I guess my number one fantasy is to be made to feel like I am utterly desired. I want to be completely ravished – for my partner to explore my body like it's a drug for them, to make me feel as if just my naked presence ignites them. Not because it's just another naked body, but because it's *me* and *my* body. Feeling so unique and hearing it from another person makes me feel desirable for exactly who I am, all insecurities aside. And the more desirable I feel I am to my bed partner, the more aroused I am.

[White American • Jewish • <$128,000 • Bisexual/pansexual • Cohabiting • No]

My sexual fantasies can include everything and anything. The only thing that is never included is me. I'm lucky to come from a country that is body-positive in every shape and form. Comprehensive sex education and open conversations about body issues made girls like me knowledgeable about our body's worth. To discuss sex was never a matter of navigating code words and metaphors, and I talked about it frequently with my friends. As I grew older, though, their experiences progressed from fantasy to real life, while mine remained the former. In discussions with them, I lied.

Whenever I fantasise about sex, the people involved will be sometimes women, sometimes men. Some don't resemble me at all. And while some of them may be close to looking exactly like me, that is fine as long as it isn't actually me. I remember for a while I created a dark-haired woman named Harriet who would replace me in every fantasy: I'd let her be taken by my crushes, my idols and my fantasies instead of myself. Whenever I came into the picture, the mood crashed and discomfort crept in. I felt disgusted.

What can be concluded from this? Maybe I just hate my body? Except I don't. I'm what the media has crowned the 'ideal' and I'm confident in my skin. Maybe I'm asexual? But I do want to have sex. I want to feel what the people in my fantasies feel. I'm sexual, so long as I'm not there. Maybe I'm scared? Of what? I've gotten the education, I've had every talk, I know how to protect myself. What am I afraid of? On the rare occasion that I allow myself to imagine my first sexual encounter, it is with a person whose face is blurred. Someone bigger than me who lays me down and takes me, gently but passionately. Someone who doesn't have to ask; they just know what I need and give it to me. Someone who makes me feel safe. Someone who doesn't make me feel like myself any more. Someone who is fine with me wishing I wasn't here. Maybe I don't think I'll ever trust another human enough to let them have sex with me like that? Not even in my wildest fantasies? Probably.

[White Swedish • Wiccan • <$19,000 • Bisexual/pansexual • Single • No]

I practise lucid dreaming. Every night I dream I have sex with the actor Pedro Pascal.

[Swiss • Heterosexual • In a relationship •Yes]

Before reading Nancy Friday's *My Secret Garden* I did not fantasise. Now, I commonly do, as I love sex but am not always ready to go; using fantasy as a tool means I can always get to a place of enjoyment. My fantasies vary and change all the time and are sometimes ridiculous and as over the top as possible. I love to fantasise about cocks, the more the better, so for example a man riding another man is a favourite (sometimes involving my partner) or many men masturbating around me. I like to fantasise that I am on a table in a banquet hall masturbating (almost like I am the feast itself) and all around me are fat, old, rich men, surrounding the table gawking and leering with their cocks pointing to the sky. All different sizes and shapes, some tiny and podgy, some large and exaggerated. They all want to fuck me.

[White British • <$38,000 • Bisexual/pansexual • Cohabiting • Yes]

In my fantasies, I'm always approached by a straight-looking older female who makes me (consensually) submit to her fully. She dominates me and uses me however she pleases. But I'm fearful of telling those around me, such as my husband or my therapist, about this. I believe there's a lot that could be said about a younger woman dreaming of an older woman around my mom's age doing those things. But since I first discovered masturbation as a high school student, it's the only thing I can think about to get to the bursting end and I have no doubt that the fantasy will follow me through motherhood and well into old age. The first time with myself was extremely difficult. Not because I didn't know how to perform, I learned very fast what felt good; I just couldn't seem to reach a climax no matter what I did. It felt like I kept climbing a hill and stopping just before the peak. This lasted for several days until I was watching a movie with an older female protagonist and realised my genitals had the ability to communicate with me. 'Bedroom. Now. Right now.' And fireworks.

I've tried thinking of my husband before, because that's what you're supposed to do, but when I do so, I'm never able to fully reach orgasm. The fantasy in my head – the woman and situations in the fantasies change constantly, depending on what TV show or movie I'm into at the time – is the only situation in which I can see myself fully allowing physical trust and I believe that's why it's the only thought that can allow me to climax. Afterwards, though, my internalised guilt is phenomenal. I stare at myself in the mirror wondering what's wrong with me and why I can't be satisfied with thinking about my husband while I touch myself. I do love him, horribly and with all of myself ... but there's a small part of me that feels like I'm missing out on the one experience that can make me sexually whole.

I did think about attempting to achieve my fantasy back when I was single. I guess there were a multitude of reasons that stopped me from searching for someone. What would people have thought if they'd found out? I'd dated women before, so that part wouldn't have been a surprise. But finding out I was sleeping with a woman my mom's age would have turned a lot more heads.

I often wonder if other women have thoughts like these, but sex isn't exactly an open conversation. I wonder if my tutors in high school ever thought about me like I thought about them. I wonder if my friend's mother in college ever thought about seducing me the way I so desperately wanted her to. I wonder so many things and I would give anything to know if someone else has these same thoughts, solely so I can know I'm not alone.

Even as I'm writing this I feel disgusted with myself. I'm not supposed to have those thoughts and it makes me want to scrub myself clean and crawl into bed with my husband. I've kept this fantasy hidden from the world and have never told it to a soul, living or dead. A part of me fears that if anyone finds out I'll be a social outcast, or possibly thrown into a facility and studied by people like Sigmund Freud. I believe sex should be an open conversation. If it was then I think there's a strong chance I could have experienced the one thing I secretly and consistently desire so deeply. For now, and until the end of my life, these cravings will stay hidden between just you and me, dear reader. I'll keep your secret if you keep mine.

[White American • Atheist • <$19,000 • Bisexual/pansexual • Married/in a civil partnership • No]

If only everyone had three lives. The first, I spend like this one, married to my best friend from school, raising our kids in the small apartment with the big tree. Our skin used to be young together. We still make love, but after three pregnancies and two kids our rhythm has changed, and that's OK because, you know, intimacy has many faces. We're like those geese, mating for life, and I'm so very grateful for the utmost sense of belonging I feel with him.

The second life, however, I spend with the unkind men, the wrong ones. The ones who touch you just this side of rough, who mix pain with pleasure, who don't really care about you. They come and go and leave marks on your body, but never in your life. Their faces change, but they are hard and big, fucking you from behind or against walls. They tie you up and tear you down, always taking more than they give, but there is a very unique kind of excitement in being taken. My second life is lonely at times, but loneliness is a choice, they say. I don't need romantic entanglements to be complete; I prefer watching geese from afar.

And the third life … the third life I spend loving her. She is wild and free, her hair a mess of wind and curls and sea salt. When she kisses me, her lips are salty as well. She has opened a cavernous space inside of me, a space I had never known existed. I'm different with her. I'm jealous and fierce and protective. I want to touch her, all the time, want to put my mouth on her, my hands. Sex with her is soft and intense and voluptuous, and she is so utterly beautiful. She consumes me like the waves of the ocean consume you, crashing over and around you with full force. And it's everything. If only. And even while living my beautiful first life, the other two still exist somewhere deep down in the candid moments between wakefulness and dream.

[White German • Catholic • <$64,000 • Heterosexual • Married/ in a civil partnership • Yes]

My husband thinks of me as a very vanilla lover. If only he knew what I dreamt of being. We're both transsexual and have difficulty maintaining a fulfilling sex life because, let's just say, our parts don't really fit us. I've taken to often giving up and watching porn while masturbating. I watch other trans women, because I relate to their sexual experiences.

I used to idolise female sex symbols, dreaming of being a *Playboy* model, and for the longest time, I've wanted to be a famous porn star. I always thought of myself as very ugly pre-transition. Transitioning really has brought out the best in me, in more ways than one. Deep down, however, I'd love to get *all* the cosmetic procedures available to make myself into a sex symbol. I've always been valued for my brains, but I want to be valued for my body. Shallow? Perhaps. But when you hate your body as much as I hate mine, you long for *anyone* to see you as desirable. And sometimes, even one person isn't enough. I want *everyone* to think of me as the very image of female sexuality. I fantasise that I star in adult films, model in the nude, am a drop-dead sexual icon. When having sex, I like to imagine myself in all sorts of risqué situations: I'm on a film set handling multiple men, or on my knees handling just one.

In real life, I keep trying to spice up my sex life, but I think it's a bit much for my husband, since he still thinks of me as very restrained. The most I've done is buy some nice lingerie and scented candles for the bedroom. I know I can't be a porn star: it would be impractical, what with also being a wife and a mother. I'll just have to content myself with filming me and my husband having sex. That's quite the turn-on, and a fuel for my fantasies at least.

[Mixed-race American • Atheist • <$64,000 • Heterosexual • Married/in a civil partnership • Yes]

I came of age during the late sixties and early seventies and met my husband-to-be when I took a government job and we were both computer nerds in the same department. I don't think it was a sexual attraction at first, rather an intellectual one. But the sexual connection kept growing through the years before and after we got married.

Fast-forward thirty-four years, and my husband died five months ago. I miss him terribly. I have been in a spouse-loss group for thirteen weeks and shared the feelings of loss with half a dozen women, most far younger than I. But no one mentioned the secondary loss of sexual relations, something that I am very conscious of. Because the sex was great, I guess, it is something that I associate very strongly with my husband's living being.

I try to recall and relive the reality and to bring some fantasy now to masturbation sessions – something that my Catholic upbringing has not made clear or simple for me – but as most widows probably would admit, nothing can really take the place of the spouse you have lost. Certainly, fantasy doesn't do very much to ease the grief. I long for touch, but I'm trying to be content with hugs and kindness from family and friends, though I remember that one of the first of those that I got after my husband died felt almost like a body blow, in that it brought home to me that I wouldn't be enjoying the full-body, *passionate* hugs I once got for a while, if not ever.

My husband wished for me to find someone else after his death – he actually told me this shortly before he died. But that is the last thing you can imagine when you have lost someone that fit you so well. I used to watch television shows and movies and think that I would love to be in a relationship with this or that actor, but I always had my real-life love to enjoy in bed. Now that I don't, I find I am easily infatuated, again, with movies and television. It's one of the things that still relieves gloom and can make me a little bit happy, particularly when the nights of widowhood seem long. I do wish there was more discussion of grief and spouse loss and sexuality.

[White American • Spiritual but not religious • <$128,000 • Heterosexual • Widowed • No]

I have been with my husband for thirteen years, married for twelve. After we got married, our sex life was pretty non-existent – not due to lack of attraction but instead due to his severe depression, self-loathing and the impact of an overbearing mother. I did everything humanly possible to encourage him to engage with me sexually: kindness, compassion, saucy underwear, talking, fantasy. But literally nothing would work. For the first five years of our marriage, we had sex maybe twice a year, and when we did have sex, it lasted for about five minutes, at most. It left me feeling empty and lonely.

In order to cope and to feel a sense of affection and love, and to reach orgasm on my own, I began to build a fantasy world. At first it began with an ex and reimagining our relationship if we had made different choices – but it just didn't feel comfortable or peaceful to me. Focusing on what might have been, what I had lost, was not enough to remove me from reality. So, I began to use books and TV, characters from movies, and it opened up a whole new world. After five years of using my fingers to masturbate, I went against my husband's wishes and bought two vibrators, and I've never looked back since.

I build the worlds of all my fantasies with incredible accuracy and in every smallest detail: what I and everyone else wears, where I live, down to what we eat. The dialogue matters, the story matters and my power in the scenario matters to me. Sometimes I'm a survivor in a zombie apocalypse: I meet someone and I save their life, we battle enemies and forage for food together. Sometimes this involves me having children I care for; my lover supports me in this role and the sexual fantasy is us fighting for each other and the survival of our family.

In another fantasy, I'm a witch in a wizarding world. I'm beautiful, powerful and able to perform magic. I wear revealing clothes which show off my body, I have sex with other wizards and witches and I'm in charge – I'm not afraid of being raped or hurt, because I can always kick the arse of any attacker. I can build on these fantasies for months, and then start a whole new one. In my fantasies, I'm free to have sex with males or females, sometimes both. The turn-on is the sexual freedom I enjoy with either sex.

In reality, my husband and I have sex maybe once a month now. We have a respectful, kind and fun relationship. He has grown in confidence and spends more time making sure I'm satisfied when we do have sex. But I find this interaction highly challenging. Part of me wants to retreat into my fantasy world but, for him, I try to stay present in our lovemaking. The level of rejection and loneliness I felt for many years, though, was incredibly destructive, and I know that without my fantasies and my fluidity in imaginary world building, I probably would have ended my life.

Women are made to believe that men want to fuck all the time; if you're lucky, they want to make love. But men not wanting to have sex due to depression, mental ill health or lack of confidence is just never spoken about. So, when you're in a sexless relationship like mine, you can feel so disgusting and worthless because you have nobody to talk to. You have a partner who tells you they love you, cuddles you, talks to you but won't be intimate with you, or when they do, they make no effort to satisfy your own sexual needs … and you have a devastating level of shame on both sides. I think that's why many of my and others' sexual fantasies involve women as the main characters; the heightened level of detail of their bodies and the prolonged intimacy that I imagine have more impact on me, because in the scenes I play out I can be more exhaustive. Many of the men I have sex with in my fantasies are deeply thorough at making me come, or they are brief entrances of cock while I'm making love to another woman. Or it's two men and me and I'm in charge and it's magical and profound. The Weasley twins from the Harry Potter films, for example. Don't ask me why, but there it is!

[White Scottish • Christian • <$38,000 • Bisexual/pansexual • Married/in a civil partnership • No]

To have my husband say he's hired a cleaner. To have my husband say he's done the grocery shopping. To have my husband say let's go to the movies. To have my husband say I changed the bed sheets and did the laundry and folded the laundry. To have my husband say your face is beautiful and not mention my forming jowls at thirty-eight years old. To have my husband say the dogs are not destroying anything. To have my husband eat me out. Then slowly touch my back, fingertips on the shoulders and along the underside of my arm and up into my scalp. To have a shaved head so I can feel that touch without having it tug on my hair. For me to be on top and find that exact perfect position which lets me orgasm (an elusive and mystical occurrence but amazing when it gets there). Then to be done from behind because a great pounding is always life-affirming. To have a bath and have double doors that open up onto a warm summery breezy garden. A fantasy. Half of it is a reality. Working so that I can make the other half happen.

[White Canadian • Anglican • <$19,000 • Bisexual/pansexual • Married/in a civil partnership • No]

Most of my fantasies involve men I have met, in person, and whom I admire. I try not to fantasise, as I am told it is a sin, and lust – as explained by Dante – does tend to leave one hanging, suspended in a state of arousal, detached from reality. Is that why I do it? I mean, my fantasies are so much more than simple sexual arousal, more than recreating the butterflies and weak knees of a first crush. I feel like fantasising gives me the will to live. I'm probably on my own with that, but honestly, if I didn't have inappropriate dreams of riding some guy like Seabiscuit, biting at his crotch to blow him, having some sexy guy hugging me for the first time ... or some girl ... I don't know that I would stay alive. I need hope. In anything, really. Even if is just plain ol' lust. The hope that one day I might have mind-blowing sex is what keeps me doing the daily grind. Sad, sinful and true.

[Irish American • Catholic • > $128,000 • Heterosexual • Married/ in a civil partnership • Yes]

Sex for me has always been a complicated subject. Abused as a child, by someone I was supposed to be able to depend on, sex as an adult has always had to involve trust. For me to want to be with someone in that way, I must feel an emotional connection. I can't just go out and sleep with someone I met at a club that night. No one-night stands for me. That's not to say that I'm not attracted to women and non-binary folks I don't know, and I do have friends with benefits. I'm also polyamorous (although currently single), as opposed to monogamous.

Sex is further complicated by the fact that I'm disabled. As a wheelchair user, I often find that women tend to think that I can't have sex – a myth we need to dispel. Wheelchair users are often just as capable of having sex as others. Although we may do things a little differently. But potential partners hear about my diagnosis of Ehlers-Danlos syndrome (in which an issue with my collagen causes my joints to dislocate regularly), and they think that sex will quite literally break me. It won't. If anything, alongside swimming, sex is one of the safest forms of exercise for me because I can communicate what works for me and what doesn't. I'm the sort of person who is confident in discussing my needs. Maybe that comes from being neurodivergent, or maybe it comes from knowing that I need to let my partner(s) know how best to prevent those dislocations, or what to do if they should happen. And if they do happen, I can usually put them back into place myself. It's not likely to stop what we're doing for longer than a few minutes at most, unless it's a severe dislocation, and those are rare. I think in part it's one of the reasons I find myself drawn to older women. They've done the work in knowing who they are and are more communicative in what they want. They respect that I know my body, know myself, and what I can and can't do. They're also less likely to see my being a wheelchair user as a notch on their bedpost. Honestly, you'd be surprised at the number of women on dating sites who will match with a wheelchair user just because they want to say they've slept with one of us. It's what pulled me away from places like Tinder and Bumble. The idea that for some women I'm nothing more than a trophy is disgusting to me. I'm a human being with just as much right to the same types of relationships as others. Yet, so many inappropriate questions are thrown the way of disabled lesbians and disabled people in general. And not just 'Can you have sex?' which we disabled people get asked, or the 'How do you do it?' question that puzzles some people about lesbians. Complete strangers sometimes ask wheelchair users about the level of feeling we have in our sexual organs; if our 'bits' are the same and function the same way as everyone else's (when no two bodies are exactly the same). Then there's the complete surprise that we are sexual beings at all. It's a minefield. I'm a disabled person with a childhood history of sexual abuse who enjoys sex as an adult. Whether it's the fact I'm a childhood sexual abuse survivor or that I'm disabled, so many people can't wrap their heads around it. They seem to negate the fact that I'm still a human being with thoughts, feelings and desires. Desires that include an older woman who sees my disabilities as a part of me and not the whole of me. One who challenges me intellectually, spiritually, physically even. One who isn't afraid to show me her vulnerability, but also who will take charge in the bedroom while still considering my physical and neurological disabilities and needs. I love taller women. I'm five foot six when standing (which I can currently do although I'm losing my mobility gradually), and most of the women I find myself attracted to are at least three inches taller than me, if not taller. I love a woman with a deep and gravelly voice, a woman with an outer femininity and an underlying masculinity. I dream of being willingly submissive in the bedroom; allowing my partner(s) to take control and truly explore my body, sending me into an enjoyable sensory overload. Of having someone who wants to explore different sides of our sexualities in a safe and caring environment. Of someone who isn't afraid to pull my wheelchair close, put the brakes on, straddle me while I'm sat in my chair and kiss me deeply. I dream of being treated as someone who is completely and utterly desirable, wheelchair or not. I also dream of a world where sex for disabled people isn't seen as taboo. Where television shows and films show disabled sex more regularly. We need more of that, and we need to see queer characters shown that way. Erotic novels with disabled characters where they aren't fetishised as well. Far too often, sex is seen as the privilege of the able-bodied. Yet we all go through puberty, and unless we're asexual, sex is something we *all* desire.

[Romany British • Unitarian • <$38,000 • Gay/lesbian • Single • No]

I have a complicated relationship with sex. I'm asexual. But yes, I do have sex, I do masturbate and I do fantasise. That might seem confusing at first, but plenty of aces (asexuals) have partners, and plenty of aces have sex. I'm one of them. Also, I'm asexual but not aromantic, which means I do not experience sexual attraction but I do experience romantic attraction. I am romantically attracted to my husband, and as I'm aware that sex is important to him, I make an effort to engage with him sexually. What this means is that, for me, when I have sex I'm rarely doing so with my own pleasure as the primary aim. It probably sounds strange, but I engage in the sex willingly when I want to, and I do enjoy it when I can be bothered to participate. It's just that, since I don't experience sexual attraction, it can be hard to get into the physical state of being ready to engage in sex, so often I'm not, to be blunt, turned on enough or wet enough to go ahead with anything. Which is where the fantasies come in.

I'm told most people have sexual fantasies, they like to picture things they'd like to do in real life, or even things that they wouldn't like to do IRL but still hold sexual excitement for them, which help them get in the mood or get off. I have those too – but, crucially, I'm not involved in any of them: I'm never inhabiting a participating figure in my own imagination. I don't picture my husband, I've never had a celebrity crush to use as inspiration, and there's no one else in my life whom fantasising about would help get me in the mood. I simply don't experience sexual attraction to anyone, so just picturing them (or things I could do to them, or things they could do to me) doesn't work for me. What I do picture is fictional characters. Usually the essence of them more than any literal depiction – if it's a live-action film or TV show I'm pulling from, I'm never picturing the actors' faces, just the characters' vibes. It's the relationship between the two (or occasionally more) that pulls me in – they have to have a certain sort of dynamic that makes me feel they understand one another completely, or would fit perfectly together in a sexual situation (often involving alcohol), or could trust one another enough to go to such an intimate, vulnerable place together. There are multiple steps to it. I'm telling myself a full story, just to get in the mood. It's a highly specific, long-winded way of getting turned on, before I'm ready to start doing anything myself.

I do this to masturbate, too. You're probably wondering about that as well – if I don't have sex primarily for my own pleasure, why masturbate? Simply put, sexual attraction and libido are different things – you can be horny without it being directed at anyone in particular. I don't masturbate very often, but when I do, I sometimes picture a pair of fictional characters, getting drunk together, getting accidentally intimate, too close and too breathless for either of them to deny that there's something other than platonic feeling going on right then, pausing in that moment, closer than they've ever been and teetering on the edge of the impossible, and then finally, finally confessing their feelings and just going for it, kissing and touching each other and getting it on – so that I can fall asleep. That's genuinely all it is for me – when my mind is too active to fall asleep naturally, I make use of my body's chemistry by touching myself until I get the sweet release of endorphins, and sleep.

All this makes the depictions of sex on TV and in films and books seem very alien to me. I don't understand one-night stands – how you'd even decide to sleep with someone you don't know in the first place, and then how you'd so easily fall into bed with them and start going at it – it just doesn't compute. Sex for me is complicated, time-consuming and only happens because I and my husband make time for it, being intimate and honest with each other, and not going too fast when my body isn't fully prepared yet. He is endlessly patient and kind, and I can only hope that everyone has that in their sexual relationships.

[White British • Atheist • <$38,000 • Asexual • Married/in a civil partnership • No]

My most secret fantasy is my boyfriend proposing to me. But this is not just a daydream, a *capriccio*: I don't just fantasise about it, I meditate about it. I would call it a 'masturtation': something between masturbation and meditation.

I start by lying down on the bed, my eyes closed and relaxed. I then try to concentrate on darkness, and imagine walking down some steps made of gradients of black; at the end of the stairs there is a door, and on the other side of the door I am in some legendary scenario I have never seen in real life but long to see. The place and the moment share this aura of mystery and beauty. And there my boyfriend smiles at me, kneels, and in trembling words poses the most wanted question. I want it lush, lavishly touching, maybe even a bit kitsch; with abundant wine, laughter and tears. At this point, sex being the most powerful embodiment of a feeling, I masturbate like crazy.

[White Italian • Atheist • <$19,000 • Heterosexual • Cohabiting • No]

I have two main sexual fantasies. In the first, I'm not me, I'm younger, thinner and I've met Harry Styles and he really likes me and wants to spend time with me. I'm usually a writer or a lawyer, very successful in my own right, and after a few dates and time spent together he starts telling me how much he likes me and wants to be with me and only me. Then it moves into very hot, sensual, passionate sex.

The second fantasy always involves my partner and another woman wanting to have sex with him. When I think about it out of the context of the fantasy, I feel it's a bit perverted and I'm uncomfortable with just how desperate she is to be fucked by him. But it usually goes something like this. He's working, fixing something in someone's house, and she's so horny. She makes him a cup of tea and talks to him. He knows that she wants him and he likes it and she is thin and wearing very seductive clothing, the type of thing he would like me to wear and look like. They start kissing and he is saying, 'No, no, I can't I'm married,' but then she goes down on him and gives him a blow job. He's really hard and desperately wants to fuck her. By this time, I'm usually near climax with masturbating. I quite often cry after I have this type of fantasy.

I didn't fantasise during sex with my partner until quite recently. He had an emotional affair with a woman, and when we were having lots of desperate sex, I fantasised a couple of times that he was fucking her. I cried after I did that also, and I'm not doing it any more. Otherwise, I never fantasise during actual sex. Lastly, I've read a lot of feminist literature over the years, and I'm trying to just be myself and masturbate in the moment. I give myself permission to be me and feel the sensations, and I never cry after I do that.

[White New Zealander Australian • <$64,000 • Bisexual/ pansexual • Married/in a civil partnership • Yes]

I grew up in a strict religious environment, which led to so much guilt and shame around anything sexual. Everything was forbidden or sinful. I began to have sexual fantasies as soon as I started my periods, around fifteen years old. I remember it vividly, as they started when I was abroad visiting relatives in Canada. We had long, long road trips and I fantasised the whole way about older boys I had seen in the school musical of *Jesus Christ Superstar* earlier that year. In the fantasies, I would be naked with them, kissing, touching, humping and grinding.

When I married, it was to a man I'd never slept with (as was the religious way). Unfortunately, I soon found out we were complete opposites. I would have sex twice a day if I could and he could happily live without it. He often made me feel ashamed for wanting sex, for wanting it too much and for expressing any desires. My fantasies became my companions from then on. Many of them would have themes of being totally free, spontaneous and wild. Maybe even naughty, breaking rules or social norms.

I would daydream anywhere about what it would be like to just go with the desire as the urge took me, not push it away. I'd often fantasise about having sex in nature. I would walk along a beach and daydream about someone taking me up into the dunes, giggling and laughing and touching until we fall into the sand. His hands push my skirt up and pull my knickers to the side and he starts licking me and holding my hips down as I hold his head. I'd imagine us stripping off and running into the sea, grabbing each other under the water and feeling so alive. Exhausted, we lie at the water's edge, letting it lap up at our legs as we make love in the wet sand, digging my hands into it as he comes on top of me. My nipples hard from the cool air, he drags his hands through my wet salty hair and makes me arch my back with pleasure as I come.

On a forest walk, I'd imagine gripping a tree trunk as he took me from behind or me on my knees on the moss and leaves of the forest floor, giving him a blow job. I don't think it is the excitement of being caught in public in the fantasy, but more the utter freedom of any place, any time. Although, while working for a theatre company, I did have fantasies about having sex with someone between scenes, hiding in the wardrobe department, in full costume. A period drama, I would be in a thousand petticoats as his hands scrambled to find my wet opening under all the layers. It would be fast and passionate as we only had minutes before being called back onstage or before being caught. Around that time, I also had a fantasy of him singing loudly into my clit to see if the vibrations would make me climax.

I feel my circumstance is ironic. I longed for sex for so long and imagined that the man I ended up with would be delighted to have a highly sexual spouse! It would be lovely to think that one day my fantasies could come true with someone. But then if they became reality what would I fantasise about? Maybe a happy sexual person can be even *more* creative and imaginative in their thinking. Thank you for this opportunity to talk on a subject which is still mostly taboo. *My Secret Garden* by Nancy Friday made me feel less alone and shameful. I hope this book does the same for many more women today.

[Scottish • Christian • <$64,000 • Heterosexual • Married/in a civil partnership • Yes]

rough and ready

'I don't want sweet and soft, I want hard and fast.'

Fantasies give us the opportunity to escape. That can mean different things for different people, and can change depending on our mood. Sometimes we may hanker for a bit of care and tenderness, other times we might want to role-play and every once in a while, we might just want to get fucked.

The contributors to this chapter write of wanting to be devoured, dominated or controlled. They want total unadulterated abandon. The letters here are about letting go, forgetting ourselves or perhaps giving ourselves, via the vehicle of fantasy, a rare chance to be entirely in our bodies and out of our heads. A place where we can give zero fucks about anything and systematically cast off our fears and our inhibitions. There is even a breastfeeding fantasy where a woman is quite literally consumed.

Given the weight of multiple concurrent demands for so many women — running a home and finances, negotiating a relationship and a busy family life — it's little surprise that there is a recurrent desire, as one contributor describes it, to just 'surrender'. They say, 'My whole body, all of me — [I want to] hand it over and let it be completely possessed by someone.' The desire to be taken, devoured, consumed is an understandably welcome relief. To be able to relinquish all aspects of the everyday and just feel. To just be a body, a thing to be used for pleasure, to be filled, to be overcome by lust. As another woman says, 'I want to be an object instead of a woman. I long to exist in this primal state. To escape from the never-ending mental load.'

In my job, I have to utterly inhabit the world of someone else (to the best of my abilities), and leave behind my own fears, desires and history. It is the very definition of fantasy. In my case, this often involves a sexual freedom (and even gender swapping) that might be too scary, risqué or even unthinkable in real life. But the safe fantasy world of my profession gives me a level of uninhibitedness without consequences that is, at times, cathartic and welcome. This is fantasy's ultimate offering: the chance to live momentarily outside of reality where rules and expectations don't exist, where we can indulge our deepest desires and submit absolutely and with unreserved abandon.

To be honest, this is a chapter to which I could contribute multitudes. My letter isn't in this section, but I identify completely with the mindset and the desire behind these fantasies. It is no doubt in direct relation to the amount I take on in my waking hours. Mother, actress, producer, writer, activist, entrepreneur — enough for many lifetimes. No wonder at the end of the day the desire to cast off everything that is on my plate (all of my own making, I might add), and be consumed by something else entirely, feels like welcome liberation. But it also somehow feels like an emotional need. Is it a scream? A primal cry that says: Help! This life of mine is full on! Take it all away for a time. Or, do these fantasies represent an equal and opposite intensity to one's life experiences? Are they a safe and uncontroversial way to salve the weight of responsibility? I've read that someone going through the menopause, for instance — when their minds and bodies are sometimes experiencing terrifying upheaval — is more likely to fantasise about BDSM than pretty much anything else. That's not my personal experience but I look forward to an increasingly rich and varied internal life as the seasons change.

•

It begins with a Dream … I find myself in a light-filled room standing before a man who seems a stranger to me. He beckons me to come to him and sit upon a stool which is facing his. He has silver-grey eyes and a beautiful, distant smile and I comply willingly to his request. Watching me, he pulls his stool up very close, wedging his knee gently and unexpectedly between my legs – we are facing each other in such a way that we almost interlock, like pieces of a puzzle. I feel exposed by this level of intimacy with a stranger, but for some reason also very secure in his presence … if not a little bemused. He looks directly into me for a long while, like he is searching for or seeing something there that is very compelling. It's unnerving – is he making a judgement? Or does he want something from me?

Then, in an accent I cannot fathom, he says, 'Pull it down.' I ask him to repeat himself and, again, he says, 'Pull it down,' but I still do not understand his words. Does he want me to untie my hair? Or pull off my jacket? Or take my top down? I feel bewildered … He smiles enigmatically, shaking his head, and says something in his native tongue, and then I get his meaning: I am to pull down the veil I had unwittingly placed over me. I can feel it – it is there, enveloping me in an ethereal isolation of my own making. I am to show myself to him. He shifts even closer to me while he speaks a language I somehow remember but do not comprehend, and begins to move in such a way that his knee presses up against my most tender self, not blatantly, but with delicate provocation. As he looks into my eyes, I realise that I *do* know this man: he is very familiar to me. With a shock I understand that he knows *everything* about me: all the things I've done and not done in my life up until now, every thought, fear and desire, every secret hope and repulsion. I find I cannot look away from his stare. It bores into me like a spotlight, leaving everything I had once sought to hide utterly open to his scrutiny. It is an intensely erotic, exposing, intimate feeling that sparks a dormant sexual longing unlike anything I've ever experienced.

He places his hands under my shirt and rests them lightly upon my waist, and begins to rhythmically move me, all the while whispering some kind of invocation, looking at me intently, smiling, and I come up against him, almost through him, we are so intricately positioned before one another. And I feel as if I am being removed from something; or something is being taken from me but being replaced by something else. This powerfully sensual exchange awakens me from the dream to find that a man is making love to me – at first, I can only feel intense pleasure as he penetrates me, but then I feel my whole body climaxing, reaching a state of sublime ecstasy beneath the weight of him. His driving masculine force moves relentlessly inside me, passionate and insistent in his urgency to give me pleasure. I try to see his face but I cannot, for there is a veil covering my own face. I feel his kisses over my cheeks, on my lips, and his tongue searching mine as he moves deeper inside me, saying my name over and over again into my ear. I am suddenly struck by his energy, so familiar once again, his essence seems to envelop me. I whisper in return, 'I know you … I know you …'

The air around us is electrified. He knows exactly how to touch me, the points of no return to lead me to, so that I am virtually powerless to regain any state of composure. He caresses the tips of my nipples with his delicate fingers. He guides my hand between my thighs and they open to his and my touch. We are moving together now in a long-forgotten dance of ecstasy, his body, his face, hands, all achingly familiar, leading me into a state of sexual bliss that brings me to tears. I know this man with all the love and desire I have ever known for any man. As I reach the edge of release, the veil slips off my face and I find myself looking into the eyes of the dream-man, only now he is real, and emanating an other-worldly light of unconditional love and compassion. His beautiful eyes are no longer the faded blue of diamonds, but are like my own eyes, staring back at me with longing. I realise that my soul is making love to me. The most astounding orgasm I have ever had originates from deep inside, radiating over my whorl of delicious nerves, through my body and straight into my heart like a jolt of life force. The merging of my masculine and feminine within carries me into another realm where I am more than the sum of my parts. I am turned inside out, completely unfolded and laid bare before my lover, my soul …

[Mediterranean South African • Spiritual • Heterosexual • Married/ in a civil partnership • No]

I want to be used. I want to be a fuck hole. I want to exist only for pleasure. I want all my holes filled. My mouth, full. My pussy, full. My ass, full. All at once, as my hands greedily grasp for more cock. I want to be fucked by strangers. I want a line of men waiting to go next. I don't care who those dicks belong to. Only that they are all for me. I want to be watched. I want an audience to entertain. A crowd to cheer as I come, again and again. I want to be an object instead of a woman. I long to exist in this primal state. To escape from the never-ending mental load. This is where I reach to when inspiration is called for. She is my release.

[Irish • Atheist • <$64,000 • Heterosexual • Married/in a civil partnership • No]

An ardent feminist. Outspoken, in control. Someone who demands equality in a relationship but whose drive to lessen suffering means a tendency to take on emotional labour to make life easier for others. Making choices, being the driving force. My God, sometimes I just want to surrender. My whole body, all of me – hand it over and let it be completely possessed by someone. No choices to be made. Just hands on the back of my neck and a solid body crushed against mine. It's tied up in low self-esteem, probably. A slight disbelief that I could be desired means I fear being the initiator – that they're just going through the motions. To be grabbed, pushed – filth whispered in my ear along with the sounds that tell me I'm wanted. It's not BDSM, exactly. The accessories don't really interest me. It's the look in the eyes of someone coming towards me that says they're willing away the space between us. Their pleasure rooted in mine. Not ticking boxes but going with the tide of desire. I must have you. I'm going to taste you. You want this, don't you? Beg.

[White English • Atheist • <$128,000 • Bisexual/pansexual • Married/in a civil partnership • No]

I fantasise about my supervisor at work. We both do maintenance at a park, which makes it easy for my mind to run wild. Doing physical labour, sweating on the trail in the summer heat, how could it not? I watch him carry heavy lumber with ease and think about how easy it would be for him to get me into whatever position he wants. He could pull me in closer to him or flip me over with one smooth movement. The sweat glistens off his forearms and I imagine him on top of me. I want to hold on to his forearms for dear life as he makes me forget my own name. His hands are strong, firm, smooth and calloused. I watch intensely as he repairs a small pipe. He puts his finger inside to feel if there is any debris, runs his fingers around the outside to clean the threads. It's like the universe is playing a sick joke on me. Internally I am screaming, 'Me! Please, PLEASE let that be me!!' His fingers work smoothly, like he's done this a million times before. I want those same fingers to carefully explore every inch of my body. I know I wouldn't have to tell him what to do to make me feel good. I catch his intoxicating smell as he walks past me or as the breeze changes direction. A combination of his natural pheromones, sweat and a little cologne. And I want to bury my face in his chest, take in as much of it as I can. His smell alone turns me on. What I would do for his undershirt after a long summer day.

I can't stop myself from staring at his lips – I fantasise about them kissing me, working down my body, sucking my nipples, building up anticipation to eating me out. I imagine his face between my legs and my fingers running through his somehow always-perfect hair. He would be ever so gentle. His lips barely grazing across mine as I feel his breath on my thighs. He'd tease me until his tongue finds every perfect spot. I want to taste myself on his lips. His voice is low, smooth and comforting. I wish I could hear all of it – the whispers in my ear, the moans of pleasure, what he sounds like as he comes. I want to hear him tell me how good I feel. I want to hear him tell me what he wants and then call me a good girl when I listen. His legs are strong and I catch myself gazing at his calves on the trail. His whole body is perfectly proportional, not one thing out of place. I want to get to know every bit of it intimately. He playfully tugs my ponytail as he walks behind me one day. My face gets hot, my body tingles and my mind explodes with new fantasies. I want him to totally dominate me. Put me on my knees, grab a fistful of my hair, and do with me as he pleases. I fantasise about him using his seniority over me. He would tell me to stay for a minute after work because he wants to show me something. Everyone would leave at the end of the day and he'd lock the door to the shop. He'd kiss my neck and start unbuttoning my shirt. I'd want him to pick me up and set me on his desk. We would frantically try to take the rest of our clothes off as we finally get to kiss and touch each other's bodies all over. As he fucks me, I'd have my legs wrapped around him, I'd be kissing his neck and telling him how much I've wanted him. He'd tell me the same. When we finish, we'd get back in our uniforms and he'd play supervisor again and tell me to clean up the mess I made on his desk.

It would become a regular occurrence, with every time just as exciting as the first. I want him to fuck me as soon as I get to work, finishing inside me. I want him to give me knowing looks throughout the day as he drips out of me. I want the rough, sweaty, fast, desperate-for-each-other sex and I also want the slow, gentle, soft love. I want to tell him I love him as he's inside of me and feel a connection like I've never experienced before. I want to feel beautiful and wanted. I want him to tie me up, tease me relentlessly, make me beg for him, and then have him stroke my hair afterwards and cuddle me until I fall asleep with my head on his chest. I want to experiment with him. I dream about trying new things I never even thought of. I want to fulfil his fantasies too. I want him to guide me, show me places on my body I never knew could feel so good.

When I fantasise about sex, I want to forget about the outside world in that moment and just think about him. I want to be selfish for once and just enjoy the physical pleasure he's giving me and not worry about anything else. I want the world to only consist of him and me, together in an intimate and passionate moment.

[American • Satanist • <$19,000 • Bisexual/pansexual • Married/ in a civil partnership • No]

I want to be fingered so hard I faint. I want to give such good head I make someone faint. I want to feel like I'm nearly dead and come back to life, but like actually nearly die, not just get a bit breathless. I want to not be able to work for a week because it takes up all my thinking time because it was *that* good. I want to feel as though I'll never feel like that again, and then have it happen again. I want it to be so vivid I wank over it for years. I also want to paint myself and my partner and buy a massive canvas and roll about on it and have sex and get bodily fluids mixed in it; spit, come, piss, the works. And then hang it beautifully in the living room, like a million-pound piece of abstract contemporary art, and everyone would feel like they had to compliment it when they came round (even if they don't like it) and only my partner and I would know how/who/what made it and we'd share a cheeky smile. The best art piece in the world.

[Romany British • Atheist • <$19,000 • Bisexual/pansexual • In a relationship • No]

Deep raw-dog anal.

[White Uruguayan • >$128,000 • Bisexual/pansexual • In a relationship • Yes]

I am a machine. I am moving rhythmically to a beat and pumping. But I am also a machine that is pumping out nutrients. I am being consumed. My lover is suckling at my teat. Another is sucking my vulva and drinking the juice. Another has their tongue in my arse. Feeding. My eyes are rolled back, we are all mindless. I'm being devoured. I am meat. I am milk. I am fruit. I'm keeping them alive. I am nothing except for this purpose. Like a sow with twenty piglets hanging off her teats. Soon I am penetrated. Their hunger has become their pleasure. They are now strong. I'm being pumped back up after giving my fluids. My lover continues to suckle as he injects. We are feeding each other now. A vulva is in my mouth. I am sucking as I am rocked back and forth, getting stronger and stronger. I am being consumed and force-fed. All of this is just how it is. We are working. We don't know why we have to do it, but we do it like clockwork and it has to be done. The thump thump of our thrusting is the beat we are keeping and this beat is crucial to our survival. Then our juices overflow. We are full. We have eaten too much. We stop pumping. We are oiled up. We slide apart. My lover and the others get up and move on. The next lover arrives. They attach to my teat and start to suck. Another arrives and attaches to my vulva. Another to my arse. They start to eat. I start to feed them. I am keeping them alive. I am being devoured. I am a machine.

[White Australian • >$64,000• Bisexual/pansexual • In a relationship • No]

Good sex starts long before a single item of clothing hits the floor. Sex is anticipation, sex is longing, sex is pain and the baring of years upon years of insecurities and desire, all bundled into an act of squeaking passion and sweat.

When I was younger, I used to fantasise about making love. I still do at times, but more often I think about getting railed. My fantasy is about losing the control I cling to in other avenues of life. It is about being flipped from corner to corner of the mattress in a manner that tells me I am irresistible to my partner. I'm straight in an abashed sort of way – I feel that I missed the boat for exploring my sexuality in my twenties and that I'll have to wait for the next round of hustings in my fifties when marriages start breaking down. But I remember watching *Borgen* when I was younger and being transfixed by Birgitte. I used to think about her coming home after a long day of politics and wheedling and fucking me on the kitchen table to the sounds of the washing machine and the light of an open fridge door. I've not really unpicked this with a therapist yet and don't particularly want to. It's an old fantasy I drift back to, at slow points in the day or just before bed.

[Chinese British • Jewish • <$19,000 • Heterosexual • In a relationship • No]

'What do you see when you look at your naked self?' – I ask myself this question all the time. Curves and flabbiness maybe but also the rawness I have. All the men I have been with loved that rawness. But it's not only about men pleasuring us – it's also about exploring and pleasuring ourselves.

Standing naked in front of the mirror, I caress myself, my perfectly round boobs and voluptuous body enriched with rawness. It gives me a boost of confidence. I throw myself on the bed and close my eyes; let go of all my inhibitions and run for the wilderness. I see his face in my mind and curl my toes. His husky voice in my head gives me shivers. I caress my body thinking of him. Getting my boobs sucked by him. Hickeys all over my body. Pinning me to the wall with one leg wrapped around his waist as he finger-fucks me with two fingers or three and kisses me wildly. Neck kisses from the back while he holds my boobs. I sit on the edge of the table and my legs are up on his shoulders as he eats me and tongue-fucks my hungry pussy. I want to sit on his face and make him eat me. God, I can't hold my wetness any more. I have to touch that pussy as he pours honey in my belly and licks it off. It drips in my pussy and he sucks it away. Just imagining this, I orgasm more than twice and squirt. God knows what will happen if anybody actually does all this to me!!

[Bengali Indian • Hindu • Heterosexual • Single • No]

For most of my adult life, I have had difficulty achieving orgasm during sex. Don't get me wrong, I enjoyed sex very much, and had a robust sex life in my twenties and thirties; but there was always that deep inner part of me that was hesitant to completely let go, to allow myself to be fully vulnerable, even with my husbands (both former and current). I always thought it was just me, especially since I can achieve orgasm through masturbation, but even then, never more than a single-climax event. When I had breast cancer and my treatment pushed me into early menopause, it was almost a relief. And then I found myself thinking of him, 'Jason', an actor in both television and film, and I felt stirrings of a longing almost forgotten.

I started going to bed at night thinking of him – his face now showing just enough crow's feet around his eyes when he smiles, his beard sporting a speckling of grey, his muscular arms still toned and looking better with age. I think about having those arms around me, feeling the warmth of his skin against mine, my nipples hard and aching for the touch of his lips. He pulls me closer, and I feel him getting bigger against me; I get so wet just thinking about this I have to touch myself. I slip my hand under my panties and feel the wetness from his touch. I am lying on my side, with him right behind me; I take my wet fingers and bring them to his lips, and then place my hand over his and guide him back down to feel how wet he's made me from his touch. I keep my hand over his, and use him to feel all of the pleasure senses he's aroused; he takes two fingers and puts them inside me, and I climax almost immediately. I feel his full hardness behind me now, straining to get free. I throw the bedcovers down, roll over, and push him onto his back, taking his boxer briefs off and standing at the end of the bed. I pull off my panties, and hop back on the bed, moving upwards over him, and pause to take in his beautiful penis. I gently cup his testicles as I take his shaft in my other hand, and bend down to take him in my mouth. He lets out a slight moan, and I take more of him into my mouth. I squeeze the base with my hand as I continue to suck on his magnificent dick. I can feel my clitoris throbbing in anticipation of feeling him inside me; I move forward again, with my hand guiding his shaft, and drop myself on top of him. Oh God, he feels so fucking good inside me; I almost pass out from that unmistakable combination of intense pleasure and pain. I know I won't last long before orgasm takes me, and I try to let him know, but I can't find my voice. He senses what's going to happen, takes off my camisole and pulls me down to him. I can feel the orgasm hit me like an ocean wave just as he holds me tight, pushes me down to the base of his shaft, and rolls us over, taking the lead on top. He feels the intensity of my climax inside of me, and stays motionless until it begins to subside. He takes my hands in his and holds me down, trying not to move too much because he knows he'll come too soon. He waits patiently, kissing my lips, my face, my neck; he whispers in my ear that it's OK, no need to hurry, he's got me. He looks into my eyes and smiles at me, for me, through me. I look at this beautiful man and want to cry tears of joy. There was no laughter or shame when I told him how long it had been since I'd had sex, how many years without any intimacy; instead he held me close, letting me enjoy his warm embrace for as long as I wanted. When I explained the cancer required mastectomies to fully be removed, and showed him the end result, there was no look of disdain or repulsion; he caressed my breast, lightly tracing his fingers over the scar and gently kissing where the tissue no longer was. I smile back at him and tell him it's OK, I'm ready when he is, and we start the final stretch of our passionate lovemaking session. He starts moving inside me, his pace achingly slow but wonderful still. As he begins to pick up speed, I get worked up all over again. I can't contain the pleasure I'm feeling from him, and I kiss my way to his ear, where I start talking dirty to him – calling him 'baby', telling him how great his cock feels inside my cunt, how much I love the way he fucks me. This gets both of us going, with him quickening the pace and me getting hotter and wetter. I ask him if my pussy feels good, if he likes the way he feels inside me, and he tells me yes, he loves how he feels inside me, and how good it feels to be with me. Our rhythms are moving in sync now, and his cock feels even bigger than before. I am urging him on, whispering in his ear how fantastic he feels inside me, and wanting us to come together. I run my fingernails up and down his back to our rhythm, and I feel myself getting ready to burst, trembling to his powerful thrusts. I can't hold on any longer, and I am consumed with the intensity of another orgasm, this one more powerful than the others. He feels what's happening to me, inside me, and revels in the pleasure of letting go, shoving himself into me as far as he can and crying out in the sweetness of his release. I know it's only seconds of ecstasy, but for both of us it feels infinite. We finally collapse into each other, completely satisfied, completely sated.

The only times I achieve multiple orgasms continue to be through the handful of sexual dreams and fantasies I have created with 'Jason'. I hope to be able to feel this passion with another person someday, but until then, I have wonderful stories to keep me company at night, and I couldn't ask for a better partner.

[White American • <$128,000 • Heterosexual • Married/in a civil partnership]

I am a firm feminist and have been for the last decade, but when I masturbate, I dream of being held down, handled roughly, called disgusting names that would make the suffragettes faint – 'cum hole', 'cock whore', 'used-up cunt'. I dream of being dominated – of being praised when I service my master properly, sucking his cock, as sluts like me should. Of being taken at any point of the day or night, with no regard for what I want. Only to satisfy him.

But it goes further than this. My deepest fantasy is to be impregnated – to be bred over and over, kept pregnant and used for nothing more than for a man's pleasure, and to reproduce. I fantasise about being milked, in milking stalls, while faceless men come up behind me and fuck me while my tits are being pumped. Breeding me, and starting the cycle all over again. It's not something I would ever want in real life, and it goes against everything I believe in and stand for. But the fantasy is so hot, I come every time.

[White Welsh • Christian • <$38,000 • Bisexual/pansexual • Married/in a civil partnership • No]

I'm a 26-year-old bisexual woman from the US. The short version of my most private fantasy is: no one has ever ejaculated inside me and I would like to experience that. The long version is: I have always had a discomfort with and fear of getting pregnant.

I've known since I was a teenager that I don't want children, and being pregnant sounds like an *Alien*-style nightmare to me. In my teens and early twenties when I first started having sex, I was always very insistent and upfront and made sure everyone was using proper contraception. Even with people I really liked and trusted at the time, internal ejaculation was never on the table. All my friends and sexual partners are aware of my pregnancy ick, but I genuinely have never told anyone, except maybe one or two really close friends when drunk, just how hot I find the idea of having someone come inside me. Fantasies are always in some way rooted in taboo, so maybe that's part of it. Even as a very pro-sex person, I feel I've always struggled with just letting go of anxiety in the moment and having fun, trusting the person I'm having sex with. With internal ejaculation, the complete abandon, the physical closeness and trust of it, the actual sensation of being filled up, are all both incredibly erotic and conceptually scary to me.

In my sexual fantasies I'm able to not be the anxious, tidy type-A person; there, I'm an endlessly charming and sexy woman who can goad others into ravishing me, tearing my clothes off, desperate to fuck me until I'm filled with them. In my fantasy, I am able to coax ultimate pleasure out of someone, watching his face flush and gripping his hair as he moans and rocks his hips and ejaculates deep inside me. Complete engulfment without any of the sort of gendered ownership we encounter in the real world. The actual mess of fluids and sweat and desperate wanting, instead of the sterile performance of sex seen in porn and other places.

Given how I feel about pregnancy and bodily autonomy in regular life, I think people would be shocked to know this about me. In some ways I've also felt shame about it because it feels like a negation of my queer identity; after all, what's more heterosexual than having sex with a man where pregnancy is possible? (Obviously this isn't true and I'm as queer as can be regardless of my sexual fantasies about men, but I digress.) This fantasy, though, transcends that, I think. It's ultimately about wanting a situation where I'm both in control and able to let go and give myself over to the raw pleasure of a situation. In the grand scheme of things, my secret is probably not all that wild and is pretty achievable on a logistical level. But it represents an entire sexual attitude that for me walks the tightrope between hot and scary, the exact delicious place where so many fantasies live.

[White American • Agnostic • <$64,000 • Bisexual/pansexual • Single • No]

My fantasies have become foreplay. Sensually speaking, they are as essential to setting the mood for sex as breathing. I am a happily married bisexual woman and I make love to my husband on a regular basis. It's always enjoyable, satisfying. But sometimes, satisfying is just not enough. It's not pleasant, tender lovemaking that dominates my fantasies. It is something very different entirely. I cannot help fantasising about someone other than my husband touching me, making me orgasm over and over again. Someone who looks at me with sheer lust and nothing more. Someone who doesn't love me. This has become my deepest desire.

It's this fantasy that occupies my mind most often. It's like a film in my head where I can press play, pause and rewind when a very specific need aches to be met. I'm on my couch in my living room with my eyes closed, naked. I spread my legs and touch myself. I'm alone but could easily be caught masturbating by anyone. The voyeuristic thought thrills me. Sometimes it's a sexy dark-haired woman walking by that watches and wants me, or the mailman delivering a package who sees me splayed wide open while his hand strokes the bulge in his trousers. Maybe it's both of them. My fingertips swoop around my clit and I moan so loud I don't hear the front door open. As soon as I start feeling bereft that it's only own hands touching me, foreign ones slide up my inner thighs to replace mine. I gasp, but my eyes stay shut. My heart races not knowing whose huge and rough or sometimes delicate and fine-boned fingers dip so deeply inside me I can barely breathe. My mouth falls open as the stranger says lewd things before they suck my hardened nipples between their teeth. At first, I want to open my eyes and look at the person making me feel so wanton, but I realise it doesn't matter who they are. Whether they're a man ready to fuck me with his fat cock, or a woman with her warm, soft pussy, just waiting for me to twirl my tongue around it, I don't care. They want me. They want me so badly I can feel it in the rough way their fingers grip my hips and their mouth claims mine. But I need them. Actually, I ache for them to yank me down, shove me to the floor, and tell me exactly what they'll do to me.

They don't ask what I want when their strong body presses against my own. As my nails bite eagerly into the flesh of their back, they simply grab my wrists and pin them above my head. I'm soaking wet when I pause my whimpering to take note of the fact that this stranger hovering above me is fully dressed while I am stark naked. I'm about to ask them to strip, when two long fingers slide past my teeth and press down on my tongue. I instantly suck them deeper, showing them just how much I want this. When I don't gag, they praise me before mercilessly teasing me with dirty talk. And God, is it titillating. I still won't open my eyes to see them looking at me with the unbridled passion I'm feeling as they touch me. Maybe it seems too much like cheating if I look up and see who's leering above. So, I don't look, because the vivid sounds of them unzipping their jeans and masturbating on top of me is the exact kind of naughty stimulation I've been searching for. I don't see them touching their sex and swirling their hips along mine. But I do feel them. Every sinful stroke.

There's noise outside now. Traffic and the voices of neighbours filter through the walls of my home. 'Let them hear you,' they say. So, I moan loudly and plead for something I'd previously thought sordid for a stranger to do. They're still wearing their shoes, for fuck's sake. Yet, I lick my lips and ask them to ride my face. They say nothing as they make swift work of unlatching their belt, snaking it through the loops and dropping it on the floor. The clang makes my mouth water. Without warning, their clothes are off and their knees straddle my neck as their dripping cunt drags across my mouth. The moment my nose nuzzles their clit, it turns into an engorged cock, expanding outward, filling my throat perfectly. Knowing someone could be witnessing our erotic act makes it even more attractive. Another voyeur watching a stranger and me pleasure one another, just feet away from the window, is so tantalising it feels forbidden. It's perfect. I give in to my fantasy fully now and spread my thighs wide. I want them to use me for their own desires. They instantly stand while my hands remain dutifully raised above my head. They're now taking full control of our tryst and leaving me no choice but to comply with what my body is absolutely begging for. And I love it. I love their hand grabbing fistfuls of my hair, the feel of their arousal leaking onto my skin, and their tongue invading my mouth. There is no love or tenderness here. There is only lust and feral desperation to fuck driving us on – the complete opposite of my usual sex life.

All of a sudden, they tug on my hair until I twist around onto my hands and knees. My cheek scrapes across the carpet as they vigorously pump into me from behind. It's rough and fast and feels amazing. Sometimes it's their thick cock that pounds into me, rattling my teeth. Other times, it is slender fingers curling and thrusting, making me moan loud enough to override the slick sounds of my sex. I'm half delirious when their come finally squirts hotly across my upturned ass. Then they push me away, leaving their mark on me, and demand that I open my eyes to see what a mess I've made. But before I can even roll over, they lean in and say, 'Such a good girl.' Then I come and come and come. And then they are gone.

I open my eyes and I'm alone again, back on my couch with my clit throbbing like a heartbeat.

[White American • Christian • <$38,000 • Bisexual/pansexual • Married/in a civil partnership • Yes]

Mostly I fantasise about passionate, all-consuming sex. Not the gentle, slow-thrusting sex, where your partner may reach down and caress your face – I want the animalistic, domineering, don't-think-just-do kind of sex, where it is just *that* and nothing else. The kind where you are being held so tight that you get red marks that may bruise, bites that hurt, but they hurt the right way as you're in the moment. Being crushed under someone's weight too. There is a form of helplessness that I struggle to explain, knowing just how strong that individual really is, how strong they *could* be, knowing that they may do anything they wish, and yet they choose not to. Having their breath against your skin that raises all your hairs and words spoken that may feel like a violation if said outside this situation; they're said in a certain tone, hushed and concealed in the moment. The kind that makes you near breathless from a mix of both shock and arousal. I want to be so engulfed in the sensations that I don't have to think about how much I can hear myself, or the creaking of the bed. I just want to feel *everything*. I want to get up the next day and be sore in a pleasant way; a reminder of what went on. That kind of sex. That is what I desire most – raw, all-consuming, passionate sex. The memorable kind.

[White Australian • Atheist • <$38,000 • Queer • In a relationship • No]

I am an open book about sex and sexuality; fluid, I suppose. I've taught my children that you love a *person*, regardless of whether they have a penis or vagina. Sex is not just penetration, though that's a great and lovely thing too. I'm a strong-minded and opinionated woman who's mostly been in control in the bedroom, so when I say the following it's not meant flippantly – I long to be ravaged by a tall German man. Made so exhausted from pleasure that I cannot stand for days. I want him to make me his all-centre pleasure zone. I have had great sex. I have had baby-making sex. But I have never had screaming-until-I'm-hoarse sex where I end up on the floor dripping from everywhere with a shit-eating grin, hoping he is just catching his breath. Know any German lads you can send my way?

[White American • Atheist • <$128,000 • Bisexual/pansexual • Single • Yes]

I don't see myself as a sexual being, as someone who can go out and get what they want, which is alarmingly disappointing. I wish I did, but as it stands I don't and I'm not sure how to. Perhaps it's because my self-esteem is low, or because I don't think I'm desirable. Maybe it's for a whole plethora of reasons, who knows. I've had sex, just nowhere near as often as I'd have liked to – and never as good as it is in my head. Rather than the perfunctory 'in-out-in-out' I've experienced with men, or the somewhat awkward, more complicated but longer, and less disappointing sex I've had with women, I want explosive, crazy, mind-numbing and earth-shattering passion. I want that sense of freeing inhibition, the hedonistic, primal, sweat-inducing sort of sex. A power struggle, a fight for dominance.

Essentially, I want someone to fuck me and get fucked back. I don't want sweet and soft, I want hard and fast; I want to tease and be teased; for pleasure to be the only coherent thought left. I'm tired of having the type of sex where I'm still able to think about how my body looks from this or that angle, or whether I unplugged my hair straighteners before leaving the house. To be honest, I haven't bothered having sex in a while because it's always been the same – I'm bored, I'm uncomfortable and I can't come. I want to be so turned on I can't remember my own name. For me, or at least in my experience, the build-up to sex has always been the best part; the tension and the flirtatious looks; the desire and the intimacy of a shared feeling that neither of you seem to be able to control. I don't mean foreplay, I'm talking about before any of that's even started.

Perhaps it's relatively vanilla in comparison to other fantasies, or maybe it's a cliché, but I want to feel as though I'm in a haze of pure sexual desire. Where the tension is so high and lust is all there is. Maybe I've met him or her in a bar or club, I don't know. It doesn't matter. But now we're in a taxi fighting to keep our hands off each other. Fighting, and losing. Their hand finds its way between my legs and it's all I can do to not rip my trousers off in the back seat. I push their hand away but I don't mean it, and they know that too, so right back it goes, higher and stronger this time. I'm so lost in want, I don't care if the driver sees. In fact, perhaps I want to be seen. They're teasing me and I'm willing, so willing I'd probably let them do anything. Somehow, we've made it to whoever's place is closest — or a hotel, who cares. We're stumbling out of the car. No further than the hallway, though, before we're tearing clothes from bodies and throwing one another against the nearest wall. I'm pinned to whatever surface I've landed against, and although I'm pushing back, there's no real force to my movements — I'm exactly where I want to be. Their hands are everywhere, my whole body feels hot, it feels electric, it feels alive. I feel alive. I'm practically writhing, caught somewhere between wanting this part to last forever and wanting to be falling off the edge. I'm so distracted I barely register that I'm being lifted and carried to the bed, or sofa — whichever it is, it's soft as I'm thrown onto it. The rest of my clothes are pulled from my body, and with what little capacity I have, I rip theirs off too. Hot, sweaty skin on skin. Nails digging into backs, hands grabbing sheets, backs arching, eyes rolling. Calling out obscenities to a God I don't believe in. Barely coherent ramblings and pleas tumbling from my lips. Moans caught in my throat, pushed out by gasps and noises I didn't know I could make. At this moment nothing else exists, just pleasure. I'm fully present in the moment. It's chaotic, it's explosive. And once we're done (and we've started again, and we're done again), I leave. I grab the clothes I can find, fix what's left of my eyeliner and walk straight out the door. I'll forget my insecurities, I'll forget their name, but I won't forget the feeling.

[*White Maltese* • *<$38,000* • *Bisexual/pansexual* • *Single* • *No*]

to be worshipped

'To have someone crave me, carnally and obscenely.'

Who doesn't want to be worshipped? To be idolised for our beauty and sexual potency? To have one's every whim instantly fulfilled, simply for being ourselves? To worship is to show reverence and adoration, and at the heart of many of these fantasies is this desire to be put first, unequivocally.

I had a surreal experience in 1996 when I was voted 'World's Sexiest Woman' by readers of FHM magazine. It was, in part, a type of worship not far off some of the descriptions in these fantasies but one I felt bewildered by at the time. I gave an interview to FHM in my cowboy-print flannel pyjamas, with an eighteen-month-old toddler nearby, having just worked a ninety-hour week. It was a time in my life when my sexuality and my identity felt disconnected, because I was experiencing, as many new mothers do, the sense of having temporarily surrendered my body to someone else that needed to come first. Being idolised in the sexual fantasies of FHM readers felt very far from my reality.

For women whose days revolve around other people, it's rare to feel like you are the star of your own show – noticed, admired, loved, desired. For them – for us – the fantasy of being put back into the centre of our own story is viscerally potent. Are the letters in this section perhaps a response to modern life for women in the twenty-first century? Women who feel pulled in so many different directions and are expected to do it all without complaint. As one letter writer says: 'I thought I'd crave something way more spectacular or unusual at this point in my life, yet finding myself caught up in a slowly collapsing marriage has left me feeling bitter, disregarded. But it also managed to reignite this deep desire to feel seen again, loved; to be devoured by someone who can see beyond me. I just want to be worshipped.' It's a simple but burning need. It's interesting, too, that 'mum guilt' is a commonly used expression, reflecting the widespread struggle of women who feel they're not meeting the expectations of society or their peers, perpetuated and exacerbated by social media. Actress America Ferrera's viral monologue in the Barbie movie aptly opens 'It's literally impossible to be a woman' and goes on to express the myriad ways in which so many women feel they are not good enough, as they battle societal norms and standards which set them up to fail.

The letter writers in this section yearn for more than just sexual gratification. There's a desire for romance to escape their daily grind, and a wish for the ultimate Hollywood ending of being the unique object of a devotional love, chosen before and above all others. This kind of 'worship' could suggest, to some, narcissism or insecurity. Perhaps an internalised fear of not being beautiful enough, intelligent enough, charming enough, not worthy of being the heroine. But this is also borne out of a deep knowledge that, for the huge majority of us, 'worship' is something that lives only in our imaginations. It's entirely out of reach and, therefore, given the opportunity, wouldn't we all choose to have the power to command undivided sexual attention and loyalty?

Which makes me think that worship is, in fact, the ultimate escape from everything that is described in that Barbie monologue; that while 'we have to always be extraordinary', we are also somehow always doing it wrong. Perhaps to be truly worshipped means to be loved, adored and respected, despite our ordinariness, and the fact that we sometimes, if not more than sometimes, get it wrong.

•

My greatest sexual fantasy is to be worshipped. I envision myself to be a goddess of some kind, just some kind of divine creature, powerful and strong and beautiful, but something more than I am now, or, at least, I want to be seen that way. I'm the Oracle at Delphi; I'm a witch; I'm a fairy-tale character, someone and something beyond their wildest dreams. I sometimes envision myself naked, or sometimes in a fantastic, long, flowing gown that's just sheer enough, but ultimately simple and subtle and sexy. There's moonlight, always moonlight in my fantasies. My partner, whoever they are, I want them to also be dressed in something simple – after all, this fantasy is about *me*. In this fantasy, I want my partner to be so obsessed with me that they can think of nothing else, like they absolutely *must* have me or they'll die. Like they sought me out, hoping they could serve me. I want to hear them beg for my attention. I want them to try to convince me they are worthy of my time. I want to hear words of praise and admiration, like they can't believe I'm even real. Their anatomy doesn't really matter in my fantasy, what gets me off is their worship, the praise, the control.

So much control that I can make my partner take the lead and still know that I am completely in charge of the situation and *everything* they do. They'll fuck me exactly the way *I* want to be fucked, hard and slow and ingratiating. We'll start with me on top, before moving on to having me on my hands and knees. I want to sit on their face and let them praise me with their tongue. I want them to be on top with my legs around them and I want to hear them moan and sigh with pleasure and say my name over and over. I want them to be focused on my pleasure and getting their own pleasure from making me come; I want it to be an act of devotion and service, but I do want them to enjoy it. In fact, I think I want them to enjoy it *too* much. I'm not interested in haste, I want it to feel slow and drawn out, trying to make the time last as long as possible, because I want my partner to want it that way. And I want them to focus on touching me, on how I feel, on getting as much of me as they can. I want passion, but I don't want anything to be rushed. A labour of love, I guess. I want their full attention and desire and them to praise me the entire time we're together. When they come, I want them to know it's because *I* let them; that it's solely because of *me*. And I want them to leave still utterly obsessed with me. I want it to feel like nothing else before. Whatever they do afterwards, I want them to know that I'm the best they'll ever have, the pinnacle of women, and I want to occupy every single one of their fantasies.

[Apache American • Pagan • <$64,000 • Bisexual/pansexual • Married/in a civil partnership • Yes]

Sometimes I think I must have different skin to everyone else. I must. Turbo skin or awake skin or sentient skin. Skin that has a bajillion neurons in every inch that can come alive and sing purely with the touch of another. I mean, if everyone felt like I did under the touch of another human hand, then firstly, nothing would ever get done, and secondly, surely we would talk about it more. Back when I was at university, I was at a meeting of the drama society, and a boy came up behind me and playfully gave a gentle squeeze to the base of my neck; the meeting came to a halt as a completely involuntary hybrid gasp-moan, loud enough to shake the walls, escaped me. From then on, everyone knew my weak spot; touch my neck and I would be pliant putty in their hands. I let them believe this because it hid the truth that it wasn't just the base of my neck. It was everywhere. Now that I'm older, I know that touch is a love language, and a way that some people prefer to be shown and to communicate affection, but for me it's more than that. I love sex, I love everything about it, but I don't understand those who can limit it to certain parts of the body, when the body as a whole is what engages in the beautiful act. Yes, some parts need to warm up, but we as a whole need to wake up. Being touched is comfort, is validation, is soulful and is sexy as hell. While I sit at my desk and write this, I draw a single finger of my own down the column of my throat and my body awakens, tingling with the ghost of sensation imprinted on my skin from last week when my husband bent me over this very desk. His front to my back, hot skin behind me and cold desk underneath. Sensation is everything. It is an awakening. To wake me up, I need touch everywhere. When I fantasise about the feeling of pure bliss, I am not even having sex. I am floating in the air, being touched and caressed by many hands, feeling every neuron in my skin activated at once, feeling my body and its capacity for sexual touch as a complete whole. Being something precious to be held, to be cherished, to be cradled and to be worshipped.

[White British • Atheist • <$38,000 • Bisexual/pansexual • Married/in a civil partnership • No]

I thought I'd crave something way more spectacular or unusual at this point in my life, yet finding myself caught up in a slowly collapsing marriage has left me feeling bitter, disregarded. But it also managed to reignite this deep desire to feel seen again, loved; to be devoured by someone who can see beyond me. I just want to be worshipped. I am often dreaming of this certain scenario which brings me back in touch with myself and my desires.

I imagine myself with a tall, not-too-handsome, but deeply attractive man: someone very masculine, but soft on the inside, with a mesmerising character. Someone who makes me feel safe, accepted and adored.

I imagine that I am standing in my bedroom; the lights are dimmed and I am undressing myself while he secretly observes me from afar. He is curious, he enjoys the magic of the little things. He approaches me very quietly and takes me by surprise. He puts his hands on my waist, and the moment I can feel his warm breath upon my neck, I start losing myself. I mostly prefer to be in control, but I love the dynamic of power play. He doesn't rush anything. I imagine him undressing me slowly, making me feel as if I am possibly the most wonderful thing he's ever laid his hands on. He lifts me up effortlessly and puts me on the bed where he takes a long time loving my body; he kisses my neck, then stops at my breasts, slowly licking them, sucking on my hardened nipples, biting them gently. (I love it when my breasts are given extra attention, it makes me so incredibly wet.) Next, he slowly moves across my abdomen, kissing my stretch marks and my freckles, and upon landing in between my legs, he makes sure to build things up gradually. He satisfies me with his mouth until I start dripping with wetness, then he inserts his fingers inside of me, and at first slowly, but more vigorously towards the end, he eats me out while fucking me with his fingers, until I reach an intense orgasm. Slightly more satisfied, I eagerly reach for his cock and start sucking him off. I just love the feeling of being on my knees, yet holding all the power. I make him very hard, but I don't let him come, because I need him inside of me first. I want it passionate and rough. I straddle him, riding him until my thigh muscles start to tremble, then I am ready for the roles to reverse, to let go completely and allow him to do the work. I imagine letting him pin me down and entering me hard, pressing on top of me, crushing me under his weight, so I almost have trouble breathing. He moves me around as if I am made of feathers and stares into my eyes as he screws the living shit out of me. I can moan as loud as I please, and the moment I start to hear those familiar wet sounds, I cannot hold back any further. I let go and squirt all over the bed, leaving it soaking wet and him wild. He turns me around for the grand finale and enters me from behind, whispering into my ear, 'You're so fucking beautiful, do you know that?' while slamming against my butt, fucking me as fast as he can, until I come so hard I pull the sheets off the bed. He finally comes all over my back and then we just lie there for a moment, wrapped together, catching our breaths while I still have to land back on planet Earth.

[White Slovenian • Spiritual • <$19,000 • Bisexual/pansexual • Married/in a civil partnership • Yes]

My fantasy is to be desired. It sounds stupid, but growing up chubby and not the best-looking, the idea that I am desirable is a true fantasy. To have someone crave me, carnally and obscenely. Having someone driven to tears by seeing me naked – a peek at my chest or even the curve of my calves in heels makes them wild. The thought of someone being so desperate for me is a turn-on; maybe it's a power fantasy. Regardless, I'd like it to be a reality.

[White Canadian • Atheist • <$19,000 • Bisexual/pansexual • In a relationship • No]

My deepest sexual desire is in dominance and worship. I want to be revered, feared and worshipped as an all-powerful goddess. There is nothing that turns me on more than a pathetic, whimpering man bowing to my every whim. Begging, pleading, desperate, aching for even a glimmer of my attention. The idea of a man thanking me for allowing him to come, or, even more, allowing him to fuck my divine body, the way that some might thank God for their blessings, is dreamlike to me.

Even more, I want to command a room. Even before any foreplay, I want my presence to radiate sexuality, power, desire, control, confidence. To strike fear and awe into a man as I enter, and then thirty minutes later to be riding him as he sweats and cries in gratitude at the opportunity, taking every order I give. I am a small, young woman from a male-dominated society. I grew up fundamentalist Christian, where any fantasy of sex was sinful, let alone a woman being anything other than submissive to one man. I feel as if I will never be able to express this part of me.

[White • Spiritual • Bisexual/pansexual • In a relationship • No]

While I know that 'the heart wants what the heart wants', as the saying goes, there's an element of my sexuality that I've never quite been able to reconcile. For context, I'm a lesbian – I love women (cis and trans), and while I'm not repulsed by men, they've never sparked a reaction in me; I'm no more likely to be sexually attracted to one than I am to, say, a rock or a tree. Similarly, I'm pretty sexually indifferent to penises, even if one's attached to a woman. But despite that, I find the idea of someone ejaculating inside me scorchingly hot. The thought that my body could please someone to the point that they lose all control, of feeling their cock throb inside me as they fill me, is intoxicating. I don't think it's a biological clock thing, either – I've never had much interest in having children, and being pregnant isn't part of the fantasy, just that being inside me feels so good to someone else that it brings them to climax. I'm fairly certain I'm not the only sapphic woman with this fantasy (I've even seen strap-ons specifically created for role-playing this exact scenario), but nonetheless it remains a puzzle to me. If I were attracted to men, it wouldn't be at all remarkable, but it seemingly flies in the face of the rest of my sexuality, leading to a strange tension within the realm of my desire. Just goes to show that brains are strange things, I suppose.

[White American • Vaguely pagan • <$38,000 • Gay/lesbian • Married/in a civil partnership • No]

The men in my fantasies fall into two categories, both common enough that I'm sure hundreds of women will write similar letters – and yet I am still embarrassed and terrified to share them. Here they are: Past Lovers and Crushes-Whom-I-Really-Liked-But-It-Didn't-Work-Out, and Gorgeous-Actors-and-Athletes-Close-to-my-Age-Whom-I-Know-I-Will-Never-Meet. The star of the fantasy changes but the plot is almost always the same. A man who I am strongly attracted to, with whom I feel safe and who genuinely likes and listens to women, shows up by chance at a bar I'm dancing in. We are both sober or have taken mushrooms – but no alcohol. He tells me he loves my hair. He smells great. He is wearing soft clothes that feel nice to brush against. That electric current passes between us – the one that tells you you're going to have sex. He asks me a few questions, waiting for me to finish my sentences, paying attention and responding to my questions for him. After about half an hour, he asks me to leave with him. Asks to kiss me in the street outside the bar, pulls me into the alley behind the bar and keeps kissing me, hands in my hair and up my skirt, holding on to me tightly but tenderly. I stop him before penetration and we walk to my place instead – which is somehow only two minutes' walk away, miraculously clean and tidy, and already lit with candles and humming with the *Dirty Dancing* soundtrack. He undresses me slowly and tells me how great my breasts, back, legs, ass, thighs are. He takes all his clothes off and stands in front of me for a moment so I can see him before me, grinning. Then he climbs on top to kiss me more and I stroke his erection with my hand. He says my name in my ear. Fingers me while he kisses my nipples and then bites my lip when I gasp. I bite back. He asks if he can put his dick inside me, and when I say yes, he braces on an arm beside me, his other arm against the headboard to push deeper into me, slow but steady. He tells me that I feel so good, that I'm so beautiful, and keeps kissing me so I almost can't breathe.

I lie completely flat on the bed and let go, until I can't think, my mind is blank, there's just pleasure. When we come together he screams my name. He doesn't hurt me or make fun of me or offer any critique of my body, or the sounds I make, or the way I move – in short, he doesn't do any of the things that make sex frightening and uncomfortable. Afterwards, he continues to kiss me and we lie there together without speaking, just smiling at each other. We fall asleep and I actually sleep through the night. In the morning he wakes up before me but leaves me to sleep. When I wake up, he holds me, brushes the hair off my face. And after I'm up and showered and teeth brushed, he wants to do it again.

Writing this has made me think of a quote I saved on my phone: 'I just want a humble, murderously simple thing: that a person be glad when I walk into the room.' (Marina Tsvetaeva, from 'On Love'.) I guess that's the common thread in all my sexual fantasies – a man I think is special who sees me as special, who is thrilled that I am the person in bed with them. Someone who is kind in general but specifically wants to be kind to me. The experience of someone liking you so much, sex is the only way to express it. Murderously simple.

[Mixed-race American • Catholic • <$128,000 • Heterosexual • Single • No]

off limits

'I cannot seem to express my secret desires to my husband.
It feels ... embarrassing and scary.'

W hat is off limits or forbidden to one person may seem perfectly permissible to another. Boundaries, taboo and shame are personal and particular, influenced by society, culture and religion. We are not born with shame, it is something we inherit or learn and its insidious reach can be felt in all aspects of our lives. As you'll see from these letters, many of them outline fantasies that might seem fairly vanilla to some, but as ever, context is everything. If you grow up in a country where homosexuality is illegal, for example, fantasies about same-sex erotic experiences will feel extremely illicit. If your religion forbids certain behaviours or desires, then they, too, will feel taboo. Yet if shame thrives in silence, then the letters in this section are roaring from the hilltops.

Only a very small number of the letters we received detailed forbidden thoughts that could be considered criminal (and those that did, for obvious reasons, did not make my final cut). But while some of the acts or behaviours described in the fantasies in this section are not – strictly speaking – illegal, they still raise questions about moral and social propriety. Some also seem to pose a challenge to the conventions of what women 'ought' to desire. It is striking that quite a few of the women in this section fantasise about a person who is just out of reach – a friend, a relative, a neighbour. The notion of 'off limits' is all the more illicit when outwardly you might have a very ordinary relationship with this person. Yet in your mind, you *redraw the parameters of that relationship substantially – and with far fewer clothes on!*

Indeed, for some women in this section, the forbidden or taboo nature of their secret fantasy is the most erotic element of the scenario: the woman who fantasies about her friend as they catch up on the sofa over a glass of wine, or another whose mind wanders to her brother-in-law during sex, instead of her husband. She says, 'I love my husband, heart and soul. Love of my life? Probably. Spark plug of my vagina? Undetermined. I'm forty now, my sex drive has never been this illuminated, and unfortunately, it's not my man that's getting me off. Technically he is, yes, but mentally my mind travels to his brother while we make love ... Wondering what he would feel like inside of me.'

As noted before in this book, fantasies have no boundaries. They do not have to conform to societal norms. They are often not hindered by the guilt, disgust or shame we might feel in our more rational moments. What is off limits is suddenly available. So we could consider these fantasies as a temporary respite from shame, an escape into a world where our desires aren't judged, however taboo. If we could loosen the chains of shame out in the real world, what new, pleasurable heights might we all be able to reach?

•

I am in love with my best friend, I want to touch her. I fuck her in my head, in my normal day-to-day.

[White British Virgin Islander • <$38,000 • Bisexual/pansexual • In a relationship • Yes]

I have many fantasies and of different kinds, I enjoy them and it seems completely healthy to me. However, there is one that may seem 'controversial' to some people close to me, being a heterosexual Latin woman and living in Latin America. It is something that I could not tell my friends, since I think they would not understand. I know there's nothing wrong with these fantasies, but culturally, sexuality is still taboo for many women in Latin America (not only same-sex fantasies but any fantasy). My husband knows about these fantasies, however, and they don't bother him.

My fantasies have to do with experiencing what it would be like to share intimate moments with a woman. What would it be like to kiss her? How is her scent? And everything that could happen in that context. These fantasies present as pretty intense, beautiful and oneiric scenes flooding my mind. In fact, these fantasies are not with women close to me: they are always with actresses, characters from movies or series that arouse my imagination – people that I see as unattainable. I don't have any sexual experience with women and, to be honest, I'm not sure how I would react to the possibility of actually carrying out my fantasy. I tried to test my friends about the 'female celebrity crush' thing to see if it would be OK to be honest with them and talk about it, as we talk about many other topics. But I've noticed attitudes and comments that do not make me feel safe to talk to my friends about the subject, thus it has been completely ruled out.

[Latin American Venezuelan • Non-practising Catholic • Heterosexual • Married/in a civil partnership • No]

My fantasy starts with myself and a friend, sitting around catching up and having a glass of wine. The kids are out for the night and my husband is away until morning. She had broken up with her girlfriend a few months back, so we have her place to ourselves. We're side by side on the sofa in her lounge, chatting, giggling, sharing stories about the kids. She leans across me to grab her glass and pauses, while facing me a little too close. We look into each other's eyes for what feels like an eternity. She leans in and gently kisses me on the lips. I'm stunned but return the kiss. My tongue touching her lips, her tongue pushing through my lips, it's a soft but passionate kiss. The kiss ends and we have an awkward moment before our eyes lock again and we fall back into the sofa kissing and touching and tearing at each other's clothes. Then we're both lying semi-naked on the floor. I move my hand down her body, touching and caressing all her curves. I gently run my fingers over her breasts, stopping to play with her nipples, they become erect and hard, I hear her moan quietly. I place my lips on her nipples and flick them with my tongue, smiling as she becomes slightly breathless. I continue to move my mouth down towards her belly button and my hands towards her hips. She lifts my head and says, 'You don't have to do anything you're not comfortable with.' I look her in the eyes and reply, 'I am excited to investigate every part of you.' I move my hand slowly down to her inner thigh. Slowly stroke her leg up towards her clitoris, gently brushing past her. She sucks in short breaths every time I am near her intimate area. This excites me and I take a deep breath. I take my fingers to her labia and kiss her in the newly revealed area, she groans. I touch her lips and begin to part them, pulling my fingers gently down the inside of them, accidentally knocking her clitoris, and she moans. When I move my fingers down towards her vagina and push my finger inside the moans become longer and a little louder. I smile, I move my mouth closer to the top of her pubis,

I kiss down towards her clitoris where I stop and flick it with my tongue. She sucks in hard and her body lifts a little off the floor. I move my other hand to part her lips and continue to tickle her with my tongue and move my finger inside her; she is wet and warm and enjoyable. I continue until she arches and lets out a scream of passion. I slow my movements and enjoy the feeling of the familiar but strange; knowing how to do this makes me feel at ease. She sits up and leans towards me, kisses my forehead and says, now your turn. She pushes me gently towards the floor, kissing and caressing my nipples. Normally I flinch when anyone touches my breasts, but I start to realise that with a gentle caring touch, I can relax and feel amazed at how erotic it is.

She continues down my body and I have a moment of body shame; three children and a very sedentary job have not left me in the best shape. She tells me to relax and that my body is perfect. She kisses down towards my knicker line; her hands move to my inner thighs. Every touch feels electric and one accidentally placed finger may make me explode. She gently pulls my knickers downward. I forget all the embarrassment about my body. She pushes me back to the floor, kisses my inside knee, and the excitement is almost too much to bear. She moves towards my intimate area, and I can feel her hair brushing me, her breath on my lips, if only she would push her lips a little closer, and when she does, I want to scream, my chest is pounding, I am throbbing like I haven't before. She gently pushes her fingers along my lips, and I let out a moan. I then feel her finger exploring me, fingers inside of me, outside of me, her tongue pushing against my clitoris. I feel like I'm about to come and she backs off, but I plead, 'Don't stop.' She moves in again, I scream a little, I'm not used to letting go, so hold back. She looks at me and says, 'Relax, no one is here, you can be as loud as you need to.' I smile and she drops her head back down towards me. She moves her tongue down through my lips and pushes her tongue inside me. I gasp. Her fingers follow, moving slowly into my vagina, no jabbing or finger-fucking, just gentle movements that send me into a heightened state. Everything feels amazing. She puts her mouth on me, pushes her lips around me and sucks my clitoris. Oh my God – I have never felt anything so good. Her tongue flicks at my clitoris that her fingers gently caress, and everything is starting to leave me. I have no control, the fireworks ignite, I'm squealing with pleasure. She seems to know everything about my body and how to make it work, and after I come a second time without warning, she leaves me with a long-lasting lick, and I shudder. She is smiling now, moving up so her mouth touches mine; I flinch but enjoy the taste of me on her. We lean back against some cushions, both a little clammy from our experience, pull a blanket across us, her arms around my shoulders. She asks if I enjoyed myself. I reply, 'The best.' I smile; never have I come so hard or felt so relaxed.

[White British • <$38,000 • Heterosexual • Married/in a civil partnership • Yes]

My fantasy is dedicated to the bricklayer who was building the new house next door with his colleague for two years during lockdown. As I was working from home, we had time to build a rapport across the wall separating my place from the building site. We would have a chat and a laugh. I made them tea during the winter when it was freezing cold; during the hot summer, I saw them with naked chests, golden skin, and brought them cold wet towels to put on their heads. I had frenzied thoughts about my bricklayer. I couldn't touch him – he was a married man. But talking to him via my kitchen window when I was having breakfast, there were few locked gazes between us. You know that moment when the time stops? He was wearing this flashy neon hoodie that I also coveted. I told him I liked it and he promised that he would give one to me at the end of his work. I was moved by the way he talked about his mum with so much love and that he sounded so happy with his wife and family. I fell a bit in love with his smile and his kindness, with his happy-go-lucky attitude. He was also into football. I have no interest in football but the way he would talk about his cramps after playing was really hot. He was simply hot. I remember staring at his bum at times. The only time we came close enough for me to feel his body against mine was the hot summer day when he came to say goodbye. That was the only time he came to my flat. I was not expecting it but as a goodbye gift he gave me his own hoodie, which still had his smell, and a giant hug. I didn't wash it for few days. I was wearing my shorts. I felt his heart beating like mad when we hugged and I wanted to squeeze his bum so much. I wanted to feel his hard-on against my peach. I wanted to know if I liked his smell, as this is a deal breaker for me. But a friend was here when he came round so nothing could happen, not even a peck on the cheek. I longed for him to kiss me passionately against my white kitchen wall.

In my fantasy it was safe to go back into the zone of the imagination where thoughts of him still turn me on. All that remains is a series of questions: a flashback of what could have been. I will never see him again. Does he think about me? Does he touch himself thinking about me? Does he think about me doing yoga in the garden in my shorts, during the autumn, spring and summer? Today, I am still wearing his hoodie and I wonder if he can feel it when I do.

[NA]

I learned this past year about the idea of limerence – placing these ideals of obsession upon unattainable people: the girl who complimented me in the subway station; the much older, straight, married professor; the best friend in high school who was in a long-term relationship with her boyfriend; the people I only know of in a parasocial context who live on the other side of the globe. I've never been in a romantic relationship or a sexual one, I've never even had a first kiss. I wonder if becoming infatuated with the unattainable is my way of circumventing the irony of being so liberated while never having these romantic connections. I figured out my sexuality in my early teens, but being an immigrant from somewhere that's not so accepting of non-heteronormative identities never let me truly be open. Part of me is stuck in a closet, unable to relate to my queer friends or seek solace in the asexual/aromantic community.

Navigating queer love and sex feels unimaginably isolating when every time I find a woman attractive, I fear that it will come across as predatory, and any time I find a man attractive, I question my own feelings, wondering if they are true or if it's the patriarchal conditioning of society. I would like to say that I don't believe sex to be a big deal and that it should exist as something unattached to connection and love. But every time I imagine what it would be like, I envision lingering touches, the softness of her skin, laughter and joy, immensely passionate kisses … all the aspects of sex that have nothing to do with the sex part itself.

My mind wanders, thinking what it would be like to be tangled in her arms, to be held in a way that gives existence some meaning for a brief moment in time. I think of what it would be like to have her lips on mine, not just as a passive act but as if we were once split in two, finally finding our way back to each other.

We'd run off on a whim to vacation in a place I could never dream of affording as we spend every waking moment alone, unable to keep our hands off each other. Her escaping her dead-end relationship and liberating me from the monotony of my life. She wouldn't judge me for my lack of experience but would show me what she likes and open my eyes to new things I didn't even know I liked. There's something so exhilarating about the idea of sneaking around, as I've always been one to follow rules. She is so far advanced in her career and I'm still relatively new in mine, but we'd share thoughts in the late hours of the night about love and life and existence till the sun bleeds through the sheer curtains and paints the room a bright orange, her face ablaze and ever so beautiful. My eyes would linger on every detail of her face until we'd eventually have to come back to the reality of the outside world and keep apart from each other outside of this bedroom. She'd return to her life and her husband and I to mine until we find moments to escape back into each other's arms once again. I think about the idea of this whirlwind romance that could only ever end in heartbreak but holds the smallest bit of hope. Whole futures of happiness and bliss and connection in the passive glances of this woman. An entire Shakespearean love story told in lingering gazes.

And I am once again brought back to reality, recognising the distance between us, that these futures will never exist. And I wonder if I only assign these fantasies of infatuation to women I cannot attain because of the irresponsibility of it, the forbiddenness of it, the excitement of it. Or if I do it because I fear true connection with others. Maybe I can't even imagine intimacy without the eventuality of it imploding because I can't imagine being loved unconditionally for me. Maybe that's where the fear lies.

[Chinese • Atheist/agnostic • <$19,000 • Bisexual/pansexual • Single • No]

In my fantasy my husband has invited his friend to stay the night as they are leaving together on a trip in the morning. After dinner, my husband goes upstairs but I pour myself a glass of wine and finish cleaning up. His friend comes in, pauses to thank me for dinner before he goes up to the guest room. By the time I go upstairs myself and get changed for bed, my husband is crashed out snoring.

I grab a hoodie and go back downstairs and into the home office, off to the side of the kitchen. I push the door to, leaving a big enough gap so I can see if anyone comes into the kitchen. I sit at the desk facing the door, turn on the laptop, and go to my current favourite porn-site address. I slip my hand down under my pyjama shorts and slide my fingers through my lips and down towards my vagina and then back up towards my clitoris. Watching the screen, I roll my finger over my clitoris. Enjoying the sensation, I put my feet up against the desk and relax into the chair. I begin to move faster and can feel myself building towards climax.

A movement in the light by the door distracts me and I pause for a moment: there's no sound, it was probably one of the cats. I resume my touch. My eyes are closed, my head is back against the chair. I am breathing heavily and trying to keep my noises to a minimum. Suddenly I hear the office door close, my heart is in my mouth, I can't see beyond the glow of the laptop so I have no idea who has joined me in the room. I hear footsteps getting closer and heavy breathing. I feel a hand on my ankle. I freeze, I look up and see the outline of my husband's friend dressed just in his boxers. I can see he is hard, and this excites me more. He lifts my leg and positions himself between me and the desk, my legs either side of him. I continue to move my hand just slowly. He kneels down in front of me, his head now in line with my hand. He can see exactly what I'm doing. He reaches up to my shorts and knickers and I sit up a little off the chair to help as he pulls them down and off, in one swift movement. His head moves close to my hand. I can feel his breath on me. He puts a hand on mine to stop me. His other hand slides a finger down through my lips and enters me, sliding it in and out. I take in a sharp breath. He presses his lips to my clitoris and flicks me with his tongue. I gasp and let out a squeal, he pushes a finger against my lips. He continues to lick and flick harder and faster and faster until I come. My hips push upward against his face and the waves of pleasure rush over me, and he continues to flick at my clitoris just enough to send aftershocks through my already quivering body. I relax back into the chair and he stands up in front of me. He has discarded his boxers so I have full view of his throbbing hard penis. I smile and then lean in and kiss its side. He stops me and lifts me onto the desk, pulls me towards him and with ease I slide onto his penis. He starts to gently push himself into me. It feels so nice to have a dick inside me, sometimes the real thing is needed. We start to rock back and forth, up and down. I feel him throbbing inside me, his breathing is heavy and beginning to get faster. I realise this is going to be quick and don't want to miss out on a second orgasm. I need to give myself a hand, so I lean away a little and slide my fingers down towards my clitoris and begin to make circles in time with his thrusts. I feel him speed up, so do I. He thrusts hard and I feel the judder as he comes inside me. I speed my fingers up to bring myself to climax. I feel the waves of orgasm coming again. I continue until it happens and l fall back a little and every nerve in my body is buzzing. I slide towards him, eating more of him with my vagina, and I can feel my muscles squeezing him inside me. We stay together until both our breathing has returned to normal and our bodies have relaxed. He steps back, kisses my forehead, then picks his boxers up and goes back upstairs. I close the laptop, grab my shorts and pull them on, then go back up to bed and settle into sleep.

The next morning when I wake, I hear my husband and his friend talking downstairs. I roll to the side of the bed and realise that I only have my shorts on. I must have left my knickers on the floor of the office. In the kitchen I grab a coffee and stand on the opposite side of the counter, next to his friend. He places his hand on my back and I feel it slide down to the bottom of my shorts and then back up the inside of them. Realising that I am not wearing knickers he looks me in the eye and raises an eyebrow, then moves his hand towards my inner thigh, lightly brushing my just bare skin. My husband is too busy making breakfast to notice. I step into the office, spot my knickers on the floor by the edge of the desk, grab them and rapidly put them on under my shorts.

Back in the kitchen my husband says he is going to pack the car for the trip. I am alone again with his friend, who puts down his coffee and walks over to me. He pushes me back into the office and kisses me hard. He slides his hand quickly under my shorts and knickers and, smiling, moves his finger over my clitoris, and I lean back against the doorway and raise my leg against the bookcase. He quickens his pace, no time to hang around. I feel the sensation building and I suck in a hard breath. I'm going to come; he can see it in my face and he lightly circles my clitoris with intent. It hits me and every muscle tightens. He holds me tight, flicking and circling my clitoris until my body relaxes. He leans in, whispers, 'Until next time,' then leaves me there, breathless and glowing, just as my husband returns to the kitchen. He has no idea of the pleasure I have just experienced.

[White British • <$38,000 • Bisexual/pansexual • Married/in a civil partnership • Yes]

One of my most meaningful sexual fantasies was born out of a frustration created by a religious dogma that I learned many years ago: in the Orthodox religion, women are not allowed to enter the altar. There are many similar rules like this – not being allowed in the church if the person is on their period or if they are wearing make-up. My separation from religion occurred simultaneously with my sexual exploration, and around that time, this fantasy was also born. Before I die, I must find an empty church – be it abandoned or not – and I want a man to go down on me as I lie on the altar and my moans of pleasure to fill the echoing room. I even fantasise that I find a young priest who is willing to do this and is not afraid that his God might punish him, as I believe sex can be one of the most religious experiences of our lives.

[Romanian • Orthodox • <$19,000 • Bisexual/pansexual • In a relationship • No]

I fantasise about being fucked in a church. In the pews, under the stained-glass windows, staring at Jesus on the cross.

[White American • Atheist • <$64,000 • Bisexual/pansexual • Single • No]

I grew up extremely evangelical in the American South so I was unaware of my queerness for a very long time (even contemplating homosexual desires would risk eternal damnation, so better not to think on it at all!). My earliest recollection of desire for an older person (in this case a female pastor thirty years my senior with a deep gravelly voice) was when I was around twelve years old. I was so drawn to her and I had no idea why. The way she commanded the stage in a time when it was quite uncommon and even looked down upon for a female to preach from the pulpit. I idolised her in a way that I didn't understand until now. I would often fantasise about her 'counselling' me in her office.

Now that I am older and an out (and married) bisexual, I fantasise about an illicit affair with a pastor's wife, or even a pastor! With the news of what happened with Jerry Falwell Jr and his wife (a story I followed very closely because it was so shocking to the community), I started to suspect that all those years of telling people not to think about sex certainly makes it even more likely that we will think about it all the damn time! I want to be 'counselled' by an older pastoral couple that turns into a throuple (just for sex, I don't want to have any other contact outside of that). I loved in the story of Jerry F. (a terrible human, I know) how he would get off on watching his wife being fucked by other men. In a way, I understand because I would also be turned on by that. I'd like to take turns with both of them and I would be their dirty little secret. No shame, just people enjoying each other's company and bodies. Since I do not believe in most of the evangelical church doctrines any more, I may have a bit of a sadistic side in that I could expose them publicly if they try to be hypocrites with their congregation, but I guess that's just my religious trauma talking …

[White American • Ex-Christian (evangelical) • <$64,000 • Bisexual/pansexual • Married/in a civil partnership • No]

When you grow up in a conservative, traditional South Asian family, you are force-fed a play-by-play of what life should look like, directly from your mother's breast milk. Girl meets boy, boy and girl fall in love, boy and girl get married, and live happily ever after. As per the South Asian parenting playbook, I nailed that exam. Now the only thing pending is babies, because heaven forbid a man and woman can enjoy each other before bringing children into this mad, mad world. See, the thing about my culture is that we don't stop to smell the roses. No, we are too busy speeding through life like a game show, rushing to tick each box and collect each win before time's up.

I love my husband, heart and soul. Love of my life? Probably. Spark plug of my vagina? Undetermined. I'm forty now, my sex drive has never been this illuminated, and unfortunately, it's not my man that's getting me off. Technically he is, yes, but mentally my mind travels to his brother while we make love. Did I mention his older brother liked me for years and I never gave him the time of day because I was hopelessly tunnel-vision infatuated with his younger sibling? Or that even after my husband and I got together, no one looked at me the way his brother did? His eyes burned into me as if he knew something I didn't. Once I became his sister-in-law, nothing changed. He never married, stared at me like I gave him oxygen, and kept a respectful distance. This didn't stop me from thinking about him while my husband was inside me. Wondering what it would feel like if my brother-in-law was in the room, watching him fuck the girl that he had loved for years, while locking eyes with said girl the entire time. Wondering what he would feel like inside of me.

[Asian Indian • Sikh • >$128,000 • Heterosexual • Married/in a civil partnership • No]

I would do anything to fuck my best friend's brother. I don't think it's healthy to want someone this much. Maybe it's a simple case of wanting what you can't have. And I can't have him. He's off limits. Tall, dark and handsome. Hung like a god, I imagine. Every day I imagine. I fantasise that I bump into him at a bar. With a bit of liquor-confidence, we begin to flirt. I can smell the whiskey on his breath. I want to taste it on his mouth. He leans close and whispers in my ear. He confesses. He's wanted me for years. I imagine kneeling in front of him and taking him in my mouth. I picture the whites of his eyes as they roll to the back of his head. His soft pants encourage me. Nothing is more rewarding than the sound of a man moaning while he's down your throat. I imagine his five o'clock shadow scratching my skin. Between my thighs. Running my hands through his hair as he devours me, completely. My back is arching. I feel it in my toes already. He's so good at it! I just know he'd be so good at it! I should feel guilty but it's not my fault her brother is so hot. And it's hard to feel bad when the things he's doing to me feel so damn good. I imagine his tongue travelling up my body. Licking my stomach, my chest. Sucking my neck – my favourite spot. When he sinks his teeth into me, my head spins. Speaking of favourite spots, I bet he knows where to find the most important one. Over and over and over again. I imagine he'd be gentle at first. So gentle and tender, it's almost emotional. But then I whisper 'faster' and he sets a new pace. And then I'm panting 'harder' between thrusts until he's fucking me into oblivion. God, I wanna be absolutely filled by him! I like to imagine us trying to keep quiet while his sister's in the next room. Why is the risk of getting caught always so thrilling? The thought of him covering my mouth while he's pounding into me makes me dizzy. She never catches us though. Our secret will always be safe. He pulls out and orders me to get on all fours. Bossy. I like it. I do as I'm told before he roughly grabs my hips and dips the front of my body down on the bed. He licks his fingers and swipes them up and down my slit until he finally slips two inside of me. He begins to pump in and out of me at a torturous pace. He knows I'm close. He can feel it. He finally grabs his cock and thrusts into me. I wouldn't usually consider myself very vocal in the bedroom. In fact, the most a guy has ever gotten out of me are a few heavy pants. But with him, I'm roaring. Every pump, every thrust is ecstasy. His sister can definitely hear us. Without warning, he flips me round and slams back into me so hard that I almost pass out. I'm coming and coming and coming. I'm screaming at the top of my lungs. He makes me see stars. He makes me forget his name. He's talented like that, I imagine.

[Filipino Australian • Catholic • <$64,000 • Heterosexual • Single • No]

For the past five years, I've had no sexual contact with another human being. Receiving or giving. My mind remembers the soft touch of her fingers; around, inside, teasing. Luring me in with her confidence. Unspoken, yet given. My body solely responds to her commands.

When I masturbate, I remember the time I unbraided my hair to let the curls tussle down. I'm there naked, her beautiful breasts now on my lips. I press her against her bedroom wall. Wasting time to get to the bed would be futile. She knew that I liked anal penetration: I had admitted this in a passing comment. The men I had been with before her were seldom, but I enjoy the fullness. That's the only way I can describe it: the wholeness of me consumed by you. Holding my arms above my head, you part my legs, lips and cheeks. I know what's coming and I trickle in delight. I never doubted the way this woman holds my wrists in one hand, the perfect manicure of the other now inside me. I am sopping for her. I always come so quickly, always for her. Squirting all over her carpet, my legs are trembling. Ferociously, we kiss. Her blonde bob entwines my brunette curls like a dessert.

My fantasy is what was once had, what will never be with her again. Uniquely ours, universally common. I know I shouldn't think about her, that's why I do. That's my forbidden. She gets me there every time.

[Mixed/Black Jamaican British • Christian • <$19,000 • Bisexual/pansexual • Single • No]

I'm thirty-three and have been masturbating to this ongoing fantasy for five years, at least. For the last three years, I have been in a relationship with a man. The fantasy has evolved with time, and I am not exactly sure how it started or how I put the pieces of the story together in my head. However, I love the type of mystery TV series that involves some high-end art, wealth and forgery, so I started to imagine myself in similar scenarios. You know how sometimes something not sexual gets you excited, and then you get sexually aroused too? My fantasy has no forgery in it, but it has wealth and high-end art. Perhaps that turned me on by itself. Then I started adding characters. It's a whole scenario that spans over time. This is the first time I'm sharing it with anyone so let's see how I go about it. The beginning and the end are fuzzy, the middle section is where I get off.

In my fantasy, I am almost myself, physically anyway, minus a few things that I have changed about my body, nothing major. I'm working for a wealthy, loving, smart, father-figure family man, in his late sixties or so. His wife is not in the story. I manage this man's very large art collection which he displays in his very large mansion … in the north of Italy perhaps. Somewhere with big villas, lakes, deep green nature, sculptures in private gardens, swimming pools, fancy patios and cocktail parties. I live in a large apartment in a separate area of the house, with an opening to a secluded garden, just for myself. This older man is someone I trust, respect, love, like a father. He is not a part of my sexual adventures. But his sons are. Two brothers. Younger one, bit of a hulk, ladies' man, warm, knows how to sweet talk and get your blood flowing faster, has smooth moves. You just want to be touched by him while he whispers in your ear, and you want to be fucked by him, hard, with his big dick, and you want to forget your name while screaming his. Then, you want him to cuddle you in his big arms. He is like a big juicy burger. You want to have fun with him. He is my sexual partner in crime. And the next morning, we just move on and get on with our lives. Until one of us knocks on the other one's door again.

I've thought so many times about when the first time I have sex with him would be. Often, I imagine an evening cocktail party which I organise on behalf of the father. Celebrating a new piece of art, which I have acquired for his collection. There is a warm breeze; I'm wearing a beautiful long silk dress. Lots of their friends and acquaintances are around and I'm being pampered by these people for my latest coup. And we flirt, me and him, with our eyes, from a distance. We take a walk to the terrace, or maybe out to the garden, somewhere away from other eyes, have some drinks. Do small talk. And suddenly we start making out passionately. Moaning, feeling each other's bodies, pressing towards each other. We can't believe it's happening. But we know that this is just fun. We are almost buddies, just with extras. However, we need to stop, get back to the party, mingle until everyone leaves. Later, we go in secret to my room. He lays me down on the bed. He is dominating, but in a measured, loving way. Reading my body's signs. He licks my body, everywhere. I lick his body, everywhere. There is no shame between us. We have loud, sweaty sex, shaking the bed, over and over again. Actually, this just plays a small part in my story.

A few weeks pass in my fantasy. With many secret encounters between me and him. And one day, I decide to seduce the older brother. He is quite different from the younger one. Both physically and personally. He is slimmer, not as ripped, just fit. Brunette, more of a serious face. More of a business mind. More of a suit kinda man. Regular-size penis. His brother has told him about me and him hooking up. He is not sure how he feels about this but I know that he wouldn't stop me if I made a move on him.

One day I bring some art documents to his office. He is stressed about his work, tense shoulders. I move behind his office chair, put my hands on his neck and shoulder to relieve the tension, alternating between applying pressure and lightly touching, asking him how it feels. He is relaxed, enjoying my touch. My hands move down towards his chest. He is getting fidgety for a moment but going along with it. I swivel his chair around, get on my knees and unzip his trousers. Confidently and looking right into his eyes, I suck his dick. He is very aroused, also surprised, a little bit shocked. But very eager. After a while he stops me and I get up to sit on his lap, kissing and biting his neck. Unbuttoning his shirt and licking his chest. I can feel him between my legs and it's making me very horny. He pushes me onto his desk and now I'm sitting on his cock. He moves his hands along my thighs, moving my skirt and my panties out of his way. Brings out a condom from a desk drawer, hurriedly puts in on and pushes his hard dick inside me. We are passionately kissing while fucking, not too fast. In a slow but steady rhythm. It's very deep. He's moving his lips down my neck, unbuttoning my shirt, licking my neck, down to my breasts. We both orgasm within a few minutes, out of breath, looking at each other, lightly kissing, not really talking in words. We know we will do it again. I get dressed and leave the room.

After a while, now that the brothers know that I've slept with both of them, I start to fantasise about bringing them both to my bed and having sex with them in various ways. Oral, anal, double penetration, anything and any position you can think of. I imagine one of them fucking me while I suck the other one. Them holding me while I have really intense orgasms. We even fall asleep on my bed, all three of us. And we keep this affair a secret from everyone else in the house. My story gets a bit blurry after this point.

Whenever I want to masturbate, I think of the first time I had imaginary sex with one of the brothers, or with both of them. Sometimes I add a bit of drama to the fantasy scenario, sometimes it's just a quick carnal act.

After a couple of years went by in real life, I started to build on my imaginary life with the art family. I think it's because I got older. My life and the lives of people around me changed in certain ways, most commonly their marital status. This was reflected in my fantasy world. I developed feelings for the older brother. He did the same for me. We didn't tell each other. Things got awkward. The younger brother noticed it. The father noticed it. And they plotted to get us to reveal our feelings for each other. At a certain point, we got married, had a child. Maybe a bit of a cliché. But, I have no sexual or any other fantasies from this particular period. Something strange happened. I started imagining the future of my fantasy's characters, including the alternate version of myself. I believe it was because the sexual part of the fantasy almost concluded upon marriage coming into play (and I am not sure why it did — perhaps because I'm not married, and I have no idea how things can be in a marriage for this version of myself). So, in my fantasy I created some drama taking place a few years in the future. The older brother, my fantasy husband, expressed his interests in having an open marriage. He thought things had become boring and wanted to spice things up. At first, I didn't want it and felt upset. After much consideration, I offered him a solution. He could go and have sex with whomever he wanted. But I only wanted to have sex with someone I knew and trusted, and this was his younger brother. He got a bit jealous but accepted it. The younger brother accepted it too. He actually had never had a relationship with anyone, because he'd always thought I was the ideal woman for him. No one else came close. And this really turned me on. So, I started having sex with him again. It was almost romantic. Like an old flame. Familiar territory but a new approach. I masturbated to a matured version of this younger brother. It was so refreshing after many years of being married to his brother and having a child with him. When I masturbated to these thoughts, I was really turned on.

Then something even stranger happened in my fantasy: I got pregnant by the younger brother. This caused some shifts in the family dynamics. Now I had two imaginary fantasy children from the two brothers, while being married to one. Sometimes my mind jumped a few years ahead again in this story. And I found myself adding more details. It feels really weird typing this, but in my fantasy, I kept sleeping with both brothers, sometimes at the same time, having a threesome like the good old days, and my fantasy self got pregnant again, not knowing and not wanting to know who the father was. At this point the version of myself was even older than the age I am now. I started wondering where this was going. It was changing from being entirely sexual, filled with wild threesomes (oh, actually, on occasion, I had a third guy: an imaginary friend of the brothers joining us in the bed), to something of a family-drama-open-marriage-soap-opera ...

I can't stop writing this story in my head, moving the characters into the future. I'm happy with my partner but we are not married, and not planning to be. And not planning on having children either. I wonder if this is my mind's way of potentially living this other life, imagining how it would be, and going wild with the scenario. I also often wonder, if, when I get older, will my characters stay the same age as they are now? Or will they also get older? How will this affect my sexual fantasy, my masturbations? This fantasy has become something so much more than just sexual in my mind. It's now a parallel, alternate self that I escape to. I'm curious to see where it will take me, or where I will take it. I'm also wondering if I'll ever abandon it entirely and write a new one. And I'm curious to analyse these fantasies in order to understand myself better, to work out what I'm trying to tell myself with their details. For now, though, I'm still letting my imagination run wild with hot sweaty threesomes with these two hot brothers. And no, I have never had a threesome in real life and I am not sure if I will ever have one. But I guess that's one thing my mind is trying to tell me, by being curious and creating these characters I feel safe with.

[White Turkish • Spiritual • <$64,000 • Heterosexual • Cohabiting • No]

I have been married for five years and have yet to reach the age of thirty. I love my husband with all my heart and our sex life is GOOD. Great even. My husband's appendage is reasonably sized, and we do enjoy using toys together, all shapes, sizes and vibration settings. But I have a desire to feel FULL. I fantasise about fisting but I am too embarrassed to ask my husband. As a woman you grow up hearing about how a vagina is no use if it's 'baggy' or 'you can fit a basketball up there'. But really, I often imagine what it would feel like. I watch porn alone and enjoy watching other people shoving large dildos or items inside their vaginas and wish I had the courage to do this too. Or even to talk about it to my husband. I grew up in a sex-positive household, nothing was taboo. But now I'm almost thirty and I cannot seem to express my secret desires to my husband. It feels … embarrassing and scary.

[White • Spiritual • <$38,000 • Bisexual/pansexual • Married/ in a civil partnership • Yes]

My most intense sexual fantasy involves my boyfriend finishing inside me – without a condom. The idea of him ejaculating inside of my vagina feels greatly satisfying because it would be *his* semen inside me and I love him very much. I know that if he were to ever cream me, that we would be sharing a mutual orgasm, as I would be orgasming instantly. I envision holding it in as long as possible before letting it drip out of me and really savouring the moment. If I am alone, this fantasy can get me off pretty fast. When we are having amazing sex together, I uncontrollably tighten up the muscles in my vagina around his penis as hard as I can, dreaming that he will ejaculate inside me. This sometimes can make sex uncomfortable for him and we have to stop until I can relax the muscles in my vagina. He knows when this happens that I am really enjoying the sex with him, but he does not know that I am dreaming of his ejaculating inside me.

[Jewish American • Agnostic • <$64,000 • Bisexual/pansexual • In a relationship • No]

I know it's such a cliché, but I fell in love with my therapist. I can't help but think of Tony Soprano and hope that I don't resemble him in any way. It's not even something that built over time: there was an immediate attraction and, as far as I'm concerned, she's Carol and I'm Therese.

The intimacy of therapy has, at times, been unbearably and enticingly arousing and these weekly sessions have contained some of the most intensely erotic moments of my life. All without even touching. Not that there's been anything untoward; she's the model of professionalism, but merely being in her presence is enough. She's a gorgeous older woman. Surprisingly she has a tiny tattoo that my eye is always drawn to. It hints at a previous life; a younger version of herself; one I'd liked to have known. She has a gentle self-assured energy that puts me at ease and I love the sound of her voice – its volume, the intonation, her accent. It's soothing and gentle but firm; she has an authoritative edge to her in the way posh English women sometimes do, and that makes me wonder what she'd be like in bed.

I love looking into her light brown eyes. She mentioned she has a cat, and for weeks after, I imagined myself to be her cat, being stroked by her, rubbing myself against her legs and miaowing. She screws up her nose when she smiles and it makes me melt. She has lovely hands, and sometimes her nails are painted red. I imagine them inside me and it gives me a jolt of desire. I wonder so much about mundane things like what she likes to eat, does she prefer to bathe or shower? What's her favourite food? Her favourite book? Music? … I have long scenarios of me wining and dining her and then fucking her.

Then I imagine that it is our last session. We get up to say goodbye and it's slightly awkward. I'm not the best with goodbyes. With a shock I see her face so close up, those kind eyes and luscious lips I've dreamt about kissing for so long, and it makes me feel quite dizzy. We hug and I hold her for longer and harder than is socially acceptable and to my surprise she clasps me tight too. A proper embrace. I've wanted to smell her skin for so long. To nuzzle into her hair, her neck. To breathe her in and kiss her and taste her. 'You smell lovely,' I tell her before boldly kissing her on the cheek. We're so close now and I can feel my heart pounding in my chest. I want her face ingrained in my mind forever and I'm worried I'll forget what she looks like. Will I be humiliated if I kiss her and it's embarrassing and awkward and will she think me ridiculous? Or will she think me a terrible lech? She's a professional doing her job, what am I thinking?!

Desire overtakes and I move in to kiss her, and to my surprise and relief, she doesn't pull back. Our tongues tentatively touch and before I know it my hands are in her hair, pulling her into me, and I start to undress her. 'I can't,' she says, which slaps me back to reality momentarily and I wonder if we have been seen. 'There's no one around, is there? We can stop if you want,' I say. But it's like something has been unleashed and this time *she* kisses *me*! I can feel the wetness between my legs. We're kissing and touching each other with abandon now and I'm unfastening her bra, trying not to be frantic but driven mad with the need for her. I see her breasts for the first time. 'Oh fuck,' I say. I take her nipple into my mouth and flick my tongue against it while caressing her other breast. Hearing her pleasure noises makes me moan with desire and I take the nipple of her other breast into my mouth. Her nipples are hard and while I'm doing this she's slowly moving her hips against me and we're pulling each other's clothes off until finally we're naked. I kiss her neck and explore her with my mouth and tongue, going lower to her belly and moving lower to her thighs. She lies down and I open her legs. To be able to see her beautiful body, and to be able to touch her, smell her and be about to taste her is more than I can bear. 'I've wanted to do this for a long time,' I tell her and take a few moments to look her in the eyes and look at her cunt. I tease her for a few moments by kissing her legs and smelling her and kissing her around her cunt, trying to draw things out for longer and have some kind of build-up, but I can't wait any longer; her smell is so alluring, I want to taste her. I put my mouth between her legs and she lets out an involuntary moan. I kiss her and then my tongue finds her clitoris and I run my tongue up and down it gently while she starts to move her hips in time with my motion and we're both moaning now. I put my tongue inside her and she's so wet and tastes just divine. I can feel my own wetness and I go back to her clitoris and we find a rhythm, she's moving her hips in time with my tongue. I use one hand to keep her lips apart and the other to touch her breasts. Her clitoris is swollen and receptive to my tongue. There's no doubt that her body is saying 'yes' even if her head is saying 'no'. I tease her with my finger at the opening to her cunt while still licking her clitoris and I can feel her body starting to stiffen and she's about to come. 'Fuck me,' she half whispers, half demands, so I put two fingers inside her and slip them in and out and this is enough to make it happen. She arches her back and cries out. My mouth is still on her and she's pushing into my face now and I can feel her cunt tightening around my fingers as I move them faster in and out. When her body relaxes, I work my way back up to her mouth with my fingers still inside her and with her cunt contracting around my fingers. I reach her mouth and kiss her and slowly take my fingers out of her and think about how much I'll enjoy having her scent on my fingers for the rest of the day. I feel elated to be lying here with her with my head on her chest and my legs curled around her. 'That was ... unexpected,' she says, which makes us both laugh and we kiss some more. I lick the sweat from between her breasts and nuzzle into her armpits, deeply inhaling her scent. We start to kiss again and this time I lie on top of her and how glorious it is to feel her body against mine! I take her hand and put it between my legs and start to move my hips and rub my cunt against her fingers and thigh. We're kissing and my thigh is pressing into her wet cunt and our movements quicken and we're thrusting against each other, our cunts wet and sliding against our thighs and we're kissing and groaning. The pleasure is beyond words. She puts my nipple into her mouth and the flick of her tongue against it, along with her fingers rubbing my clitoris and our sounds and motion, makes me come fast and loud. She leaves her hand between my legs as my wetness covers it and the muscles of my cunt contract around her hand. We lie for a while, our bodies entwined. We kiss and start to move our hips in time with our thighs moving against our cunts again. I want to feel her cunt on mine so I move into position and we're both so wet and it feels so wonderful and to be able to look into her eyes while doing this is a bonus. We hold hands for leverage and grind against each other cunt to cunt, she's so soft and wet, and listening to her noises I know I'm about to come and I tell her I'm going to and she pushes into me and she's now going to come too. We're both moaning as we orgasm at the same time and we're both well and truly spent.

But in a few minutes, we've arranged ourselves decently and we lapse back into our roles as if nothing had happened. And, of course, it hadn't – apart from in my wildest fantasies.

[White British • Atheist • <$64,000 • Gay/lesbian • Single • Yes]

the captive

'My heart is pounding, I'm terrified, but the way he touches me is like something I've never felt.'

*I*n our real lives, safety and consent are foremost when it comes to sex. In fantasy, however, things can stray into dangerous territory, as the contributions in this section show. Many of these letters came with caveats and justifications like 'I've grappled with this fantasy a lot. It's a sexual script where I am not in power and it's bothered me.'

I thought long and hard about including some of the fantasies which featured more violent scenarios, including those describing being held captive and engaging in sex with a captor or captors, because these could be interpreted as rape fantasies. I am very conscious that this is a highly contentious subject. It goes without saying that the last thing any of us wants is to normalise any form of kidnapping or violence towards women. Yet omitting these letters and denying the fact that many women do fantasise about such things feels disingenuous and could potentially breed the shame this collection seeks to break down with open and honest representation.

But what does it say about women, for whom sexual assault is an ever-present fear, if they fantasise about being captured and ravaged, often not only by one man but by many? I am not qualified to comment about the psychology behind certain sexual proclivities, or the role of such fantasies in our imaginations, but what I can say, with utmost certainty, is that very few women would want these particular fantasies to play out in real life. Erotic thoughts of being overpowered and held prisoner by a violent assailant are about sex. Sexual assault is about power. And in a fantasy we, the women, are uniquely in control of what is being done to us. We are the director in our heads; we make the choices about how our bodies are treated. Obviously, in real life, the reverse is true. We are powerless.

Sexual fantasies about being ravished are of course about power and control, but not in the way we might assume. In a fantasy of being coerced or held captive, the woman is necessarily playing the submissive role. But her fantasy is also about controlling her partner. As the one in charge of the direction of the fantasy, she is the puppet master, the one who has reduced her sexual partner, be they a stranger or a known loved one, to such a state of sexual arousal and desire that they cannot control themselves. This also plays into the idea that these fantasies are borne out of a need to be so intensely desired, to be seen as so irresistible, that their sexual partner loses all sense of restraint or decorum.

Many years back I played Dr Bedelia Du Maurier, Hannibal Lecter's psychiatrist in the TV series Hannibal. In one season, Bedelia is held at Hannibal's Italian palazzo, where his excess and depravity are on full display. She can leave but she chooses to stay. Is she under his coercive control or is it her choice? Is she turned on by the danger? The fact of her captivity is arousing bordering on erotic – it's almost like a fever dream made manifest.

A word of warning: the following fantasies do contain descriptions of sex that blur the lines between consensual and non-consensual. So while fantasies allow us total creative control, the same is true of your reading experience. You, as readers, have a decision to make; you have the choice to read these fantasies or not, and the decision is entirely your own.

•

The fantasy I have the most intense reactions to is one that goes against many of the things I value, and I used to feel very guilty about it. It's simple, really: I lie in bed, alone, and a bunch of men enter my apartment. I don't see them, I don't know how many there are, and yet I know they're all obviously perfectly my type. Sometimes they're burglars, other times they lost their way right into my place and took the opportunity. Said opportunity, of course, is to have their way with me. They blindfold me before I can see any of them. Really, I'm a nuisance to them. They're not here for me, they're here for the fun or the valuables or whatever, and at first, they overlooked me still being in the house. They don't mean to rape me. But I'm naked and in that bed and one of them is tasked to make sure I don't make a peep to make their life miserable. So, on goes the blindfold, a hand around my mouth, another to keep me still, a few more in the room to make sure I don't cause trouble. Then it's usually my moaning that gives it away, or sometimes one curious man among them, who 'can't help' but look and touch, will notice the state I am in. This is how they notice how wet I am. How sensitive I am to every touch and brush. How much this is turning me on. They'll brush their fingernails across my nipples and recoil in surprise at how wantonly I react. And then there are more hands, more than I can count. Building tentatively and getting bolder and bolder. Touching, probing. Other voices joining in, telling my guests to cut it out, this is not what they're here for. 'But look how she wants it,' they'll say, or something like it. It will just be a little bit more. And more. Just five more minutes. Just one more touch. 'I'll just rub my cock here a little, look how she bites her lip for it. I'll hit her clit with it like so, look how she moans. I'll put in just the tip.' Because they can't help themselves either – I'm turning them on, too. They're as hard for me as I am wet for them. The first slide into me is accompanied by a broken moan that is not my own but that of the person I envelop and suck into me. He didn't mean to do this, but he couldn't help himself. This was not his plan, but here he is, his cock sliding into me after all, even if he promised his buddies he wouldn't, that geezer, he could control himself, don't worry.

This, the imagination of him finally breaching me, is where I'll be rubbing myself and come directly. No frantic pounding, no double penetration, no nothing. Just the image of a bunch of faceless attractive guys spell-cast by my desire, attracted to me, and one of them entering me with one deep, slow and lustful stroke only, while the others' hands are on me, is all I need to come. Even writing this, I'm soaked wet and yet I haven't touched a single part of myself. I've grappled with this fantasy a lot. It's a sexual script where I am not in power and it's bothered me. It's dubious consent at best and that's bothered me, too. But I am the one who writes this story in my head, over and over, and it's not reality but I am the director, and God I want it when I dream it, and so I definitely consent to it. This fantasy is nothing I would want to live out for real – it could not have the quality and safety it does in my head. At best, I would want it in a safe and consensual play scene – something I would never dare to enact. I am a feminist. I'm sex-positive. I'm powerful and have a lot of responsibility and sometimes that is stifling and I want a break from it and to let go. I'm monogamous and happy in my relationship. And I've embraced this fantasy as my own, my private place; nothing about this fantasy is wrong to have.

[White half-Jewish German • <$38,000 • Bisexual/pansexual • Married/in a civil partnership • No]

My fantasy is one I have shared to a degree with my best friend. We have created many such shared fantasies over the years, with characters and ourselves as characters in these long-form daydreams, and speak frankly and openly about the sexual details, too. We've created versions of my main fantasy together many times over the years, but the details of this one below are all mine.

I have somehow been caught by a group of incredibly attractive biker men, who are holding me captive at their base. They taunt and tease me initially, enjoying my frustration as I struggle not to admit I fancy them all very much … One day I do something to anger them, however, perhaps attempt an escape, and that's when the fun begins. The group of three to five biker men surround me, nearly letting me run off but always catching me, tearing my clothes off one by one. Eventually I am fully naked and very turned on, as are they, and they guide me down to suck on all their cocks, one after the other. They are impatient, grabbing my head or my hair, and thrusting into my mouth. The activity builds, with them all touching my body and using my mouth for their pleasure, until they want more. I am laid down, and they take turns to fuck me. They do not simply use me, though, they also make sure to touch and pleasure me, teasing me for how much I clearly enjoy it. However, at some point I manage to slip away from them again, and now the mood turns from gently teasing to the need to punish me. They bend me down over the bed, feet on the floor but my upper body on the mattress, and their leader spanks me. With my ass sufficiently red (and my pussy very wet), he then thrusts his big cock first into my pussy, and then he spreads my buttocks. He rubs his cock between them, letting me know what's about to happen before he starts to work his cock into my ass. I struggle but it is not painful: deep down, I love being taken anally, too. Each of the men fucks me in the ass, some slowly and enjoying every bit, others faster and rougher, delighting in the gasps it elicits from me. If I resist, they simply kick my legs open wider and grab my arms, holding me in place and open for them. At this point, they bring out a vibrating wand, placing it on my clit and attaching it with something so I can't escape the sensation. They continue taking me this way all night long, through multiple orgasms and ejaculating inside all three of my holes.

[White Finnish • <$38,000 • Bisexual/pansexual • Single • No]

My fantasy, which may sound disturbing, involves travelling abroad and being kidnapped by a terrorist organisation. OK, just to clarify: I do not support violent organisations. I do, however, come from a background of childhood trauma where the threat of violence was very real. I have shared a house with a murderer and a paedophile. Whether that trauma played a part in creating this fantasy, I am not sure. But in my fantasy the kidnappers have to be very dangerous. They hold me hostage, interrogate me, I am scared. I plot my escape and lie in the foetal position on a very dirty and uncomfortable floor. Eventually one of my captors comes into the room and grabs me by the hair to ask why I am not eating the food they left for me. I don't answer but we make eye contact. His one hand stays put with a firm grasp on my hair, the other starts gently sliding up my body, over my dust-covered trousers and then under my baggy T-shirt revealing my soft skin. His hand stops when it reaches my chest. My heart is pounding, I'm terrified, but the way he touches me is like something I've never felt. I don't know his name, we don't speak the same language, but he kisses me and takes off my clothes. The sex is very passionate and not violent in the slightest. We tease each other, kissing and then pulling away. He holds my hands above my head and interlocks fingers with me. I can feel each drop of sweat from his face falling onto mine. But every time our eyes meet, I still see the same look as during my abduction – violence, pain, a need to destroy in his eyes. Therein lies the fantasy, being passionately fucked by someone, seemingly caring about me and my body with every action they make, while their eyes tell a different story. I can't stop looking at his eyes. Seeing the power and darkness in him makes me more turned on. I know he is a dangerous person, but I've never felt more connected to someone. The way we read each other's bodies shows respect and love. I look into his eyes one last time and see the anger, the danger. I come. I'm not sure if he does or not. He gets up, opens the door and motions for me to leave. Outside, the street is loud and crowded. I look back at my captor and his eyes haven't changed. I shudder. Is this really happening? Am I free? I blend in with the crowd and start walking away quickly, before he changes his mind. I'm free. I'm empowered. I'm lost.

[Hispanic/White American • Taoist • <$38,000 • Heterosexual • Cohabiting • No]

Growing up, I remember that my first (chaste) fantasies as I was falling asleep at night involved me being injured or disabled in some way, and then nursed back to health by a mysterious nebulous figure. I don't know where I got my inspiration. Maybe I watched *An Affair to Remember* at a much-too-impressionable age? Maybe it was just always there?

Later, as I got older, the fantasies became less chaste, and the mysterious nebulous figures sometimes less kind, a captor rather than a saviour and often vaguely sexually (and sexily) menacing in ways I couldn't always define. I'm in my forties now, queer, polyamorous, semi-disabled, no longer an innocent small-town kid. My fantasies have gotten rather more explicit too. But the core of them has remained solidly the same.

In my fantasies I am never in control. I'm injured and incapacitated and in need of care, or I'm tied up and menaced in some way. In my real life I'm a big fan of consent. In my fantasy life, my consent doesn't matter, and even better, it's not necessary. Everything that happens to me, no matter how taboo, is both something I want and something I don't have to ask for. It's freeing in a way sex can never be with my real-life partners.

[White American • Episcopalian • Bisexual/pansexual • Married/ in a civil partnership • No]

kink

'I'm usually real open with friends about what turns me on, but there's one thing I don't tell anyone …'

S *ex is a subjective experience. While we are always, as humans, keen to categorise and label, it's clear that one person's kink is another person's vanilla.*

Tentacles, door handles, hairy armpits or adult nappies, the world of kink is a cornucopia of passions and these letters are a window into just a small corner of this ever-expanding sexual universe. As a working definition, kink could be considered a broad term for consensual sexual activities that are thought of as 'unconventional', whereas a fetish is sexual desire linked to a subject, an object or non-genital body part. No matter how fantastical, supernatural or 'strange', all fantasies are a product of the marriage between our direct experience – what we've seen, heard, smelled, tasted, touched – and the expansive creativity of our imagination.

We all use the word 'kink' in our everyday speech without any sexual connotation – the kinky curl in someone's hair, a twisted wire, a painful kink in your back. The logic of the word assumes that there is an objective 'straightness' to all things, and indeed, our understanding of 'kink' in the sexual world defines desires and preferences that sit outside what's considered conventional or normative. Yet the very suggestion that there is ever any standard norm when it comes to sex is lunacy. And I only had to cast an eye over the 'Dear Gillian' letters to see that there is a limitless spectrum for sexual activity, desire and fantasy which actively resists rigid and obvious classifications.

The selection of fantasies here are the ones that surprised me the most. Not because I am a prude or easily shocked (trust me), but because the extent of the wild creativity and expansive imaginations completely exceeded my expectations. From the woman who is repeatedly aroused by bumping into a door handle and another who gets excited by the 'vulnerability' of hairy armpits, to those who find eroticism in period sex, bloated bellies, wearing diapers and sex with tentacles – these letters are testament to the extraordinarily wide-ranging powers of invention of the human mind.

In the fifty years since My Secret Garden, *the range and diversity of kinks and fetishes have changed and expanded. The power of technology and the accessibility of the internet to much of the world enables easy one-click access to Google searches for porn sites on every conceivable kink manifestation or specialist interest, no matter how niche. Moreover, the internet has enabled communities to build around particular kinks and fetishes, meeting at clubs, parties and even at dedicated conventions – a literal bottomless resource that modern women can draw on to explore and articulate whatever arouses them most.*

And yet despite all this, and the fact that popular culture features sex that revolves around kinks more and more, and that research shows BDSM is second only to group sex as the most popular of all sexual fantasies, the shame society casts on kinks persists. It's hard to know what percentage of these fantasies ever get voiced or realised, given so many women still feel fearful of judgement. But thankfully it seems that our rich imaginations – especially when they feature kink and fetish – are increasingly uninhibited.

•

I bumped into it on my way into the office, and instantly I was attracted. It started with slight brushing of the hand to full-on grasping it in its full glory. The door handle: I would sneak in after hours to pleasure it to its full extent. My husband didn't know, of course, but he couldn't provide me with what I needed as a woman, the full girth and stretchiness I experienced with this partner.

[Jewish • >$128,000 • Have intercourse with any object, person or thing • Married/in a civil partnership • Yes]

I like my men hairy and emotionally vulnerable. Just a brief glimpse of a hairy belly, revealed when a guy's shirt rides up, gets me fantasising about taking his clothes off and getting my lips all over his body. When I close my eyes and go to my happy sexy place, I fantasise about kissing a hairy man's chest and belly and thighs all over, or lying against his warm chest as he fingers me, or feeling his hairy belly sliding against my body when he's on top of me. I'm usually real open with friends about what turns me on, but there's one thing I don't tell anyone: men's hairy armpits *really* excite me. It's about the vulnerability because, seriously, armpits are several different kinds of physically vulnerable. It's also straight-up about how they look. The contours of armpits are gorgeously complemented by the presence of hair. Guys doing pull-ups can be like porn for me. Mostly I just love to look but sometimes I think about kissing them, like I end up fantasising about kissing every other hairy body part I find sexy. Dicks make me feel all 'Oh yeah, I get to play with that' and asses are 'I want my hands on that' – but if a guy shows armpit, 95 per cent of my attention goes there. My brain short-circuits and I'm stuck thinking, 'Oh God, oh God, oh God, those are his armpits and they are right there, being all hairy and beautiful and incredibly sexy and look at that, LOOK AT THAT!'

[White American • Atheist • <$19,000 • Aromantic, mostly sexually interested in men but occasionally people of other genders • Single • No]

Period sex, whether it's heterosexual, lesbian or somewhere in between. There is something very raw about having sex on your period. It's messy and it's natural. It's sweet and 'nasty'. Something so stigmatised I believe can bring people closer together. To fall in love with a person even when they're bleeding and cramping. To find beauty in the ability to bear children. Period sex is hot. It's fun and it tastes good :) I love it.

[White • Buddhist • <$38,000 • Bisexual/pansexual • Single • No]

When masturbating or when I'm having sex with my husband, I often imagine a kind of penile tentacle moving towards me and then penetrating me. It will then withdraw and then penetrate me over and over again. It is often, in that magical way of fantasy, coming from below me and managing to get between my tightly closed legs. It's normally quite slim and somehow lubricated. Also, it's not embodied – it's just a questing alien thing. It's not seeking pleasure, it's just curious. I never give any thought to what this tentacle-like thing is attached to. I just need to imagine it searching me out and entering me repeatedly.

The other thing that gets me really hot is imagining myself breastfeeding adults, mostly men. They suck greedily and really enjoy my milk, or are just peaceful and contented. With my second child I had far too much milk and had to ask my husband to relieve me. I was so engorged it was more a physical relief than a sexual pleasure. But I often return to that memory and make it sexual, or imagine feeding some other cherished person in my life. It makes my pussy tight just thinking about it.

[Married/in a civil partnership • Yes]

I wet the bed deliberately almost every night, and I love it. It is so liberating for me – the freedom to pee wherever I want and in whatever way I want; it took over a year to fully commit to it, and I've never looked back. Wetting myself fills me with confidence, but also with the desire to be controlled. It extends beyond just my bed, too. I love to pee in my trousers, skirts, shorts or sometimes just my panties, sometimes in my bed or on the toilet or even in my car! I also enjoy wearing and wetting pull-ups, little training underwear for girls; they make me feel small but also confident. The first time I wet myself in them I had the best orgasm I ever had up to then; they held all my pee too as I have a small bladder. I have a few pairs of panties and pull-ups in my purse with me at all times, in case of an unfortunate accident while out of the house.

My fetish really took off for me when I went away for college. I had my own dorm room and bathroom. I could indulge any time I wanted, which now could play into my second major fetish: flushing my panties down the toilet. I don't know what I find so sexy about it, but I now do it in a safe manner in a way that cannot affect anyone other than myself. I'm not even connected to the public sewers, so no worries there.

I'm still a virgin and wetting, pull-ups and flushing play heavily into my fantasy of how I want to lose my virginity. In my fantasy, my bedwetting is discovered by my lover, who then comforts me while I cry in my wet panties or pull-ups, telling me that it's all OK, accidents happen. They help me out of bed and take me to the bathroom to clean up and dispose of the evidence of my bedtime accident. This becomes a daily occurrence. I wet the bed every night with my partner, who even teases me about my accidents, maybe almost telling their friends that I wet the bed. Humiliation sometimes plays a part in my fetish depending on what mood I'm in. Sometimes I want to be in charge; other times I want to be protected and cared for. Sometimes I feel invincible to the world, other times I feel the need to be protected.

[White American • Christian — non-denominational • <$128,000 • Bisexual/ pansexual • Single • No]

I have had many a fantasy over the years. Some have died, others have developed and the desire for them to actually happen has grown stronger. They are things I cannot entirely explain. One relates to a fetish I have. Most would call it breeding, although there is another term, 'hucow'. I cannot speak for all that it encapsulates, but, in short, I really enjoy the idea of being 'filled'. I don't even know if I can explain the extent to which I desire it, that sensation of feeling someone finish internally right against the very back of me and all that comes after (the semen slowly leaving me, having it run down my thighs, too). If there was a way to have a man never run out of semen, I would probably never wish to leave the bed, wanting more and more. The thought alone is enough to stimulate me, and it often occupies my daydreams.

[White Australian • Atheist • <$38,000• Queer • In a relationship • No]

My biggest sexual fantasy is a very niche kind of pet play. Instead of a pup or kitten, I prefer to play as a black leopard. Sure, I wear the ears and the tail that most expect, but I also wear a pair of sharp-clawed gloves. It's a grey area between dominant and submissive, being a pet with a sadistic streak. This dynamic is empowering to both myself and my girlfriend. The pet knows it is capable of violence, biting and scratching and playing a little rough. The mistress knows this too, and keeps the beast in check while letting it use its talents. Sometimes I fantasise about guarding my mistress at the foot of a throne, lounging at her feet. Other times I wonder what it would be like to be ordered to hunt another submissive at her command. Being told 'sic 'em' and being let off my leash.

[White • Atheist • <$19,000 • Gay/lesbian • In a relationship • No]

I have known I was transgender since childhood. When puberty kicked in and I was both feeling a strong sexual drive and experiencing more gender dysphoria from the masculine changes I was experiencing, I started to develop fantasies of not only being with a woman as a biological woman myself but also about women peeing on themselves. I'm not sure if this started because the diapers symbolised a way to cover up my maleness or if it was a traumatisation from wetting the bed until seven years old and the shame I was made to feel from it. Either way, lesbian or girl solo pants-and-panties-wetting videos became my go-to porn. Sometimes even diaper-messing videos if I was drunk.

I developed a very strong AB/DL (adult baby/diaper lover) identity as well as my not yet admitted female and lesbian identity. When drunk, I asked my exes if they'd still want to be with me as a girl. They all said no, but I could close my eyes and could pretend I was being eaten out by them while receiving oral sex. It was my only outlet. Also, I did have my exes wear diapers for me because I am extremely attracted to girls in diapers. Adults, of course. But now that I have come out as transgender and AB/DL, it has not only freed me from my pain and suicidal ideation but I can finally live my life through my own eyes instead of living through my exes and my fantasies. I am so happy to say I found an amazing fiancée who loved me as male but stayed with me as female and gets turned on by the diaper stuff as well. Believe it or not, only one of the many girls I've ever introduced to diapers wasn't into it after trying it. They all were hesitant at first but they loved it so much after wetting for the first time. It is so sexual and I think all girls should try it because it's not something we expect to enjoy, but I can tell you they do. I can't wait to have my surgeries and I dream about the day I can finally experience the ultimate desire to be fucked by my lesbian girlfriend while I am the one finally in the diapers. Nothing turns me on more. I am so happy with my ability to finally admit to the world my gender identity and my sexual interests.

[White American • Christian • <$19,000 • Gay/lesbian • Cohabiting • No]

In the last decade or so, my sex life has been very intermittent, but my fantasy life is rich. I have an ambivalent relationship with blood. I would be extremely reluctant to have a blood transfusion, for example, unless it was from someone I was either related to or very close to. And yet I fantasise about blood exchange with someone I was deeply in love with. Just imagining it is very intense and highly erotic for me. Blood is one of our most potent fluids. I guess there is a reason why vampires are sexy, Gary Oldman as Dracula in particular. The scene towards the end of that film when Winona's character drinks of his blood, mmm. I also have a vague recollection of watching a French movie – a young woman's sexual odyssey – roughly twenty years ago. In one scene, the protagonist is bound and blindfolded, sitting on a bed. A man cuts her knickers with sharp scissors just at her vagina; he then inserts his fingers through the cut cloth. Around the same time, *Secretary* came out. Both of these movies opened me up to the idea of submission.

When I think about sharp surgical scissors, and the feel of the cold steel on my skin, cutting off clothes, I get hugely turned on. Recently I started fantasising about being cut with a scalpel. Being bound and controlled, and cut on various parts of my body – small neat cuts, drawing blood – then blood exchanged, licked, swallowed, then cleaned up and Steri-Stripped. (All with the full understanding of the requirement for clean health re: blood-borne diseases, of course!)

[White European • Atheist • <$64,000 • Heterosexual • Single • Yes]

Ever since I was a child, I have been turned on by girls' bellies that are bloated from eating too much. I remember watching my belly expand when I would eat a lot and it gave me this sensational feeling. Of course, now I understand it was arousal! Where and why did this become a fetish? Girls' bellies in particular are the source of arousal even today. It's not in the 'traditional' realm of kink so I am very shy about it, despite being involved in a kink community where no stone goes unturned. This fetish just feels 'odd' compared to the other more mainstream ones.

My fantasy would be to have a big dinner with another girl, maybe a guy too. Afterwards we go to bed and play with each other. I always imagine myself sitting with my back to the chest of my partner, with them leaning their back to the wall. Their hands rubbing my belly and kissing my neck as I drink water to bloat some more. Partner number two would be eating me out at the same time. And BOTH would make me feel normal and loved and cared for in all this so I'm not self-conscious that I look fat or unattractive to them in my bloated state. I'd also like this scenario reversed. A girl sitting and leaning back into me, my legs either side of her and my back against the wall. A guy eating her out and me rubbing her bloated belly as she drinks water, allowing herself to get bigger. I'd also squeeze her thighs and love handles.

I told one partner about this fetish once, but nowadays I keep it to myself or just minimise it to: 'I like my belly being touched and rubbed.' Meanwhile, I get really horny after eating dinner with them and they have no idea it's because I'm bloated, and not from the romance of dinner together – but that helps too. I've also been turned on by a cute bit of gluttony. When someone eats too much and burps a little and is moaning they are so full. THAT gets me. I spend Thanksgiving with my friends. You can only imagine how difficult this occasion is for me being surrounded by my attractive friends, drinking wine and feeling frisky the entire night from everyone's full bellies. It's a HARD day. This is all different to 'feederism', but there's something about that temporary overindulged state that I desire SO much.

[White British • Spiritual • Bisexual/pansexual • Single • No]

I'm in my late twenties, a point in my life where I'm starting to know what I like, but there is still so much to find out. Two things you should know about me: firstly, my friends describe me as kinky. Secondly, I don't like vampires. It will be obvious why the latter is relevant later. But to the former, I feel blessed to grow up in a country where talking about sex isn't taboo, it's actually pretty common. I love to explore, to get to know how my body feels and how that changes at every point in my monthly cycle. Not just the hurting nipples and cramps, but also what's going on inside my head. Apparently, some women can get horny around the time of their ovulation. But we don't necessarily talk about what we *feel* and *think* during our period.

Most of the time, my fantasies are much the same, sometimes about the soft sex between lovers, sometimes something a little more exciting – bondage, flogging, a little anal action. When I get my period, however, that all changes. There is one more thing you should know: I hate blood, especially if it comes out of my body. I put a tampon in, eat too much ice cream and hate everybody, until I notice that I'm suddenly super horny. And then the same fantasy pops up in my head.

I'm in a room without any windows. On the floor, there is a burgundy velvet carpet (I don't care who cleans it afterwards, it's my fantasy). There are Victorian chairs in every corner and a dark wooden table in the middle. It is surrounded by metal frames, big enough for a person to stand under. The party starts when the single door opens and two women enter, wearing blue-and-black brocade corsets. One might describe their profession as dominatrix, but today we shall call them 'chaperones'. They are followed by eleven women whose Venetian masks obscure their eyes but can't hide their excited smiles. Since this fantasy occurs frequently, I like to change my role in this scenario. Today I'm one of those masked ladies. Some of us have been here more often than others but we all love to come back. We are all dressed in different costumes: corsets, dresses, a leather suit; one of us is wearing only a belt around her naked hips. All our outfits, bar one, have this in common: our breasts and pubic area are fully exposed. The chaperones strap ten of us into the metal frames, our arms above our heads, our legs spread wide. My skin starts to tingle, my body feels as if there is a fire burning inside. The eleventh woman has to wait. She is in the long Victorian dress, the one whose delicate parts are covered. It's her first time at the party. This night is going to be her initiation rite to join our little society and she will give something as a gift.

When the chaperones finish strapping us others up, they turn towards her. They lay her down at the table in the middle and fasten her arms down beside her body. She closes her eyes and smiles. I imagine she is as aroused as I am. I definitely was when I was lying there at my initiation. But I'm glad I can watch her. (As someone who loves both men and women, it's very arousing for me to just imagine seeing other women naked and vulnerable.) The door opens for the last time that night. In comes a group of men wearing brocade vests and dark coats, their faces also covered with Venetian masks, and they are rocking white stockings and buckle shoes: Victorian vampires. And suddenly, vampires are the sexiest creatures I can imagine. Of course, they aren't real ones, they don't have any fangs and they survive sunlight, but they are men pretending to be vampires. Now the rite begins.

The vampire leader steps forward holding a goblet filled with red wine. While he murmurs a prayer chant in an unknown language, the chaperones open the lacing at the front of the initiate's dress and pull it apart. As her soft breasts appear, I see the men's trousers stretching around their hips. The young woman looks nervous as the chaperones pull her skirt up to her stomach to reveal her already soaking-wet vulva. Each places a hand under one of her thighs, lifts it up and they push her knees towards her chest, spreading her vulva wide open. The head vampire stops his prayer and places himself in front of the woman's spread genitals. He sets his goblet aside on the table, then, without a warning, he pushes his thumb and index finger into her vagina and feels around. She starts to moan in pleasure. It takes him a while until he pulls out a piece of golden metal, formed like a small cup. It holds all her menstrual blood. He raises it a moment, then he pours the viscous liquid into the goblet. His fingers are sticky and red. Now blood starts to drip out of her vagina onto the table. The head vampire raises the goblet into the air and the others start to cheer as he takes a sip. He passes the goblet on to the next man. In turn, each of them drinks from the goblet. Now, the rite is over and the party starts.

While the men watch, the chaperones walk through the room and proceed with us like the vampire did with the woman in the middle. They push their fingers into us, grab the small cup und pull it out, slowly of course, we don't want to miss any pleasure. Finally, when it's my turn, the chaperone woman smiles at me. She knows me, I've been here a few times, so she isn't so gentle any more. She just sticks her fingers in; my vagina stretches and then I sense that warm, sticky liquid oozing out of me, running down my thighs and dripping onto the carpet. Now all the men are walking around the room, every one of them picking a woman. One of them comes up to me, looks at me smiling and then kneels down. He grabs my legs and sticks his tongue into me. I feel how he laps my blood, how he licks every drop of it from my thighs and my labia. Just a moment later, the room is filled with moans, from me, from the other women and the new girl in the middle.

Once again, I remember being in her position. Thinking about being watched by everyone, being the centre of attention, only increases my arousal; meanwhile the guy between my legs intensifies the pressure of his tongue on my clit. My muscles are getting hot, ready to contract as I'm coming. But right at the moment where I think I'm ready, he stops, leaving me with unbearable tension. I have a small break, then the next guy approaches me. He's moving elegantly and he is very polite. I bet he won't be nice at the end when he won't let me come. He proceeds with me like the guy before did. He kneels down and starts licking me, very slowly and softly. It feels like torture. I want him to fuck me, I want him to give me more.

I look around. Everyone is sharing my experience. I see their lustful faces and the men who are kissing them everywhere. Then I take a look at the woman in the middle. She is currently being entertained by a vampire man with long hair. I watch her closed eyes, her red face, her moving chest. I see how his big dick moves in and out of her asshole while she is moaning louder than all the rest of us.

'Fuck me,' I say to my vampire guy. I can see his eyebrow lift behind his mask as he looks up to me, his face full with blood. I do have to ask him. We are here to be drunk. For everything else we have to give them our permission. So, I beg him. He smiles, saying, 'As you wish.' Then stands up, rubs his bloodied face with his sleeve and gets his dick out.

'Not like that,' I say. 'Like that.' I look to the woman in the middle.

His smile widens. 'As you wish,' he repeats.

As he walks behind me, his hand touches my breasts. Then he pulls my butt cheeks apart and rams his cock into my ass. I needed no warning – I am ready and my butt hole sucks him in. He pushes his cock in so deeply, I can feel the tip pressing against my womb and his balls on my butt. Then he is thrusting, hard and deep. He lays his hands on my nipples and presses them in. Just a few thrusts more and I feel like I need to pee. I feel desperate, I just want to climax. The urge to pee gets stronger and suddenly I feel a lot of liquid squirting out of me. Every muscle in my body tenses and I can finally come.

I open my eyes and I am back in my bedroom. I smile at my partner who lifts his head up from between my legs and smiles back. I am perhaps confused by what I just saw in my head, get myself under the shower – and go back to being a blood-hating feminist who tells guys what to do instead of being dominated.

[White Austrian • Raised Catholic but not religious • <$64,000 • Bisexual/pansexual • Cohabiting • No]

My mother died when I was thirteen. She took it upon herself to teach me as much as she could as she knew her end would be early. I remember her teaching me about circumcision, penises and, of course: 'Make sure your man cleans underneath that skin.' She taught me how to pull back foreskin with a pencil and paper around it. It was all so strange when I was young. My curiosity was strong to know what a penis looked like, how it grew. In elementary school, we all had to do a project on a bodily system. I naturally picked the male reproductive system.

Once I reached maturity I realised penises are just beautiful. I am also very good at washing and pleasing men in the shower. Thanks, Mom! I don't think men know how much us women love penises sometimes. This brings me to my fantasies. I have told my partner this fantasy and we have experimented with it a bit. I love the look of a peeing penis, it turns me on. Something so masculine about it. Also dominating, which I love as well. It's something I don't share with the average Joe and was always too scared to tell anyone before my current partner. Pissing, I'm into pissing. I'M INTO MALE PISSING! Nerve-racking but also satisfying.

[Guyanese Canadian • Atheist • <$128,000 • Bisexual/pansexual • Married/in a civil partnership • Yes]

It's been a while since I'd gone out without my baby. It's nice being able to run errands alone. However, today is taking a lot longer than I'd anticipated. My breasts are full of milk and starting to ache, my bra more and more uncomfortable with every minute. I try to tell myself that it won't be much longer and, looking around to make sure no one's watching, I quickly slip my bra off, hoping to buy a little more time. But as I find the last few items I need in the store, I can feel that familiar hot tightness that tells me my breasts are too full and about to release. I dump my basket of shopping on the checkout counter hoping to make it out of there in time. Too late. Wet spots start to bloom on my shirt. Shit. 'I'm sorry, do you have somewhere I can go to take care of this?' I ask the young man at the till. Without hesitating he locks his register and says, 'Follow me.' He leads me to the 'mother's room' at the back of the store. By the time we reach it, milk is dripping from my shirt. Embarrassed, I ask the shop assistant to hold my items for me while I get myself straightened out. 'Of course, but before I go back up front, perhaps I could help you,' he offers. I'm shocked. 'What do you mean?' I say. He apologises for being so forward then says, 'I can see you're uncomfortable. Hand-expressing enough milk to make you feel better will probably take a while. Besides, they're probably pretty sore. Sucking on them won't be as painful in the beginning.' I think about it for just a moment and reluctantly agree. He is right, it would take ages to express manually and it would hurt. I sit down on a chair and take off my sodden shirt. Milk immediately spurts forcefully from my nipples. The man kneels down in front of me and takes a first nipple in his mouth. He sucks on it perfectly. Hard enough to release the pressure in my pounding breasts but gentle enough not to cause any pain. After a few minutes I feel much better. The breast is still full but no longer hurts. Then, horrified, I notice that the man has started rubbing himself.

'What are you doing?' I yelp. He stops sucking on my nipple. My milk is still flowing, leaking down my belly.

He says he's sorry, he didn't mean to embarrass me, but sucking my full breasts has made him so horny and his cock is so hard it feels like it's about to explode. He thought he could just come in his trousers without me noticing. He says we can stop if I prefer.

I pause. The pressure is already building up again in my breasts. I still need help so I tell him to carry on.

Then he asks me if it would be OK if he took out his cock and relieved himself while he's relieving me. I understand how he's feeling. I'd been so desperate I've let this strange shop assistant suck on my tits, after all. Milk is still seeping from my nipples. 'Do what you need,' I tell him.

He unzips his trousers and exposes his very hard, very thick cock. I'm frankly amazed at just how big and thick it is. He takes my nipple in his mouth once more and begins to suckle while he pumps on his prick. I try not to stare but his size is impressive. I start to get aroused as I watch him jack off, while he greedily gulps down my flowing milk. I try to squeeze my free tit so milk will land on his cock but my aim is off. Finally, I speak up: 'Would you like me to spray my milk on your cock?'

He almost comes right then at the thought of his cock covered in my milk but he manages to contain himself. 'I would love that,' he tells me. I squeeze on both my tits and milk showers over his throbbing dick. He carries on pumping away at his cock and sucking on my tits and I becomes even more aroused. I start to wonder what his cock would feel like inside me. Then I ask if he wants to come inside me.

He releases my breast as he lifts up my skirt. A drop of milk trickles from my nipple. He pulls my panties to one side and slowly slides his thick cock inside me, filling my pussy. I can feel every movement he makes. When he begins to thrust deep into me, it hurts a little but not in a bad way. In my heightened arousal my milk starts to flow heavier again. He takes a breast and sucks long and deep. Milk sprays into his mouth and onto his chest. With that, he explodes inside me, his cock throbbing as he comes. I orgasm too and my pussy tightens around his cock. Come drips from me. He continues to suckle my milk until it finally stops flowing. He doesn't want to waste one drop.

[<$128,000 • Heterosexual • Married/in a civil partnership • Yes]

strangers

'Has this man noticed me at all? If our shoulders touch the next time the train brakes to a halt, would he feel the same excitement as I feel in my stomach?'

A ll of us have walked past an intriguing stranger on the street and done a double take. We've sat near someone on a train, or spied someone from afar in a bookshop or at a party who inspired our sexual fantasies. We know nothing about them; they could be a horrible person in reality, but sometimes a mere fleeting glance is enough for our imagination to run wild. One letter describes an experience that will be familiar to many of us: 'The train is packed. Sweaty and tired bodies are all strewn together as we all try to get to our destinations. These people with whom I never even make eye contact, let alone strike up a conversation, flow through my mind: thinking about what their names are, fantasising what our lives would be like together.' It's an archetypal storyline that's been hugely romanticised by popular culture: the thrill of catching a stranger's eye, making a connection and spontaneously following them into the unknown is the stuff of countless books and films.

So I was not surprised by the number of letters about the stranger fantasy. But what exactly is so alluring about the idea of having sex with a total stranger? Is it the surge of lust that accompanies a lingering glance, injecting some unexpected eroticism into a morning commute? The sense of anonymity, perhaps – they know nothing about you, which creates a blank slate where you can write a new, exciting identity, liberated from your daily domestic woes. Or is it the tension created by being in a public place, where any sexual arousal must necessarily be contained? There's something oddly intimate about sharing rituals with a complete stranger — waiting for a bus, a film or a takeaway — and feeling their hot gaze on your body.

And then of course there is the simplicity — it's the ultimate expression of 'no strings attached'. The intrinsic anonymity means any attraction is purely physical, without the added complications of personal details or potential relationships. Fantasising about a stranger represents an opportunity to step off the treadmill of first dates or finding a partner, to instead seek satisfaction in the here and now — no questions asked.

In the opening episode of a series I starred in some years ago called The Fall, my character Stella Gibson, a celebrated detective superintendent, propositions a young detective on their first meeting. In every interview I did after the first episode aired, journalists would ask me about that scene. Even now, a decade on, I still get asked about it. Clearly people were intrigued. But they were also shocked. The gall! Women envied her, men lusted after her. But what became clear in the media's overreaction was that the scene, only ten years ago, was indeed the stuff of fantasy.

As women, we have been rightly taught to fear the allure of the attractive stranger; the promise of seduction or sex with a stranger could spell life-threatening danger. But in fantasy, that risk is thrilling, and seems to encompass, however counter-intuitive, a sense of safety. In these fantasies anonymity is protective: a stranger exists without any of the baggage that comes with knowing someone too well. Strangers can join us for a single moment of pleasure where we are in complete control or gratefully under someone else's. For the contributors fantasising here, the mystery inherent in anonymity brings a powerful erotic force.

●

I am at a clinic designed to help people orgasm. I check in for my appointment and am asked to disrobe, sit on a table and put my feet in stirrups. Someone enters the room to let me know that in order to get to the good part, I have to be clean. They very gently give me a sponge bath, describing everything they're doing to me as they do so. Afterwards, a male doctor moves me to a bed, and asks me to describe what's happening and why I can't come. As he listens, he trails the back of one finger up and down my vulva comfortingly. When I'm done talking, he asks me if it's OK if he rubs my clit to see if I can get wet. I say yes and he does it, telling me I'm a good girl when he feels the first bit of wetness. He is very encouraging, and asks permission before every single thing he does. This continues until he pauses and looks down; he is very hard. He says, 'I'm so sorry, my penis is so hard that it hurts and I won't be able to continue unless I address this. Do you mind if I touch myself for a minute?' I do not mind this, and watching his hand move over his hard cock, I'm getting more turned on and I touch myself. He gets harder and harder until it seems to become unbearable for him, at which point he asks me if I'd be OK with him being inside me until he comes. I give him an emphatic yes and he starts to put the very tip of his dick inside of me, but I am so turned on that he doesn't get all the way in before I have an enormous orgasm.

[White American • Spiritual • >$128,000 • Bisexual/pansexual • In a relationship • No]

I'm picturing the very crowded morning tram on the line to the university. Sometimes they don't even open the doors because there are too many people, but if they didn't the scenario in my fantasy wouldn't work.

I've been instructed to get on at the far end of the tram line, for my usual stop. There are lots of free seats but I don't sit down. I stand where I've been told to stand, at the back near the doors, and hold on to the bar. The tram reaches the city centre and more and more people get on. It gets busy, then crowded, then packed. I'm waiting for someone; some man I've never met before. He's meant to get on at the main square but I don't know if he will. Sometimes I fantasise that it's raining outside and people's wet umbrellas are brushing against my bare legs – I'm not wearing any tights, even though it's cold. No knickers either, because I was told not to over the phone. The tram is warm and humid, smelling of coffee and morning breath and sweat. Over the tannoy the woman announces the various stops. This is my tram, my city, but in my fantasy I'm new here and not sure where I'm going.

I'm still holding on to the bar at the back of the tram. We're really packed in now. I keep being jostled by people's rucksacks; my face is near someone's armpit, stinking of Lynx; there's a baby crying further along, but I can't see it. I can't see much above chest height. In real life I'm taller. It's weird because I speak this language, but here and now I don't.

The tram is crawling, stopping and starting, and people are falling against each other. Someone drops their coffee down someone else's shirt. I hear angry voices but understand nothing. Coffee runs across the floor and touches my shoes. That's when I feel the hand on my hip. I look down. It's a big grubby man's hand, fingernails bitten down and dirty. It looks strong. I can feel the guy's breath against my scalp but I don't turn round to look because the not-seeing is part of it. Maybe I couldn't turn even if I wanted to. The tram really is very full now. I am looking down in fascination at this hand, which goes under my skirt and stroking the tops of my thighs. I'm nervous and excited, because this is how I have been told it will go. He's rubbing himself against me as I stand there, pressed tightly against him. His jeans are dirty, with paint or plaster on them. I can't get away because there is no room to move, so I have to stand there and let it happen. I feel the hand moving, hidden by my skirt, and now it's rubbing against my clit and I really can't do anything about it, so I just squeeze the handrail I'm still hanging on to and try to part my legs a bit.

The people all around us are looking at their phones. They have no idea what's going on here. Then this man I can't see must have unzipped his jeans, because suddenly it's not just his dirty fingers carefully rubbing but a whole rock-hard penis thrusting into me. It knocks the breath from my body because I really wasn't expecting it, even though that's why I got on the tram in the first place. It hurts. I'm trying not to make a sound, even though it's so much to take and even though I'm certain he's tearing me. I'm knocked off balance, gripping the bar white-knuckled as the tram moves and stops and more and more people fall against me. I blink down at the floor as this faceless man ejaculates inside me. He steps back, zips up and disappears. I think he's pushed his way off the tram. The floor is black linoleum and I can see splashes of semen on it, dripping down from me. Before I have time to think clearly, I feel another set of hands on my hips and another erection pressing into my back. That's when I realise I hadn't understood the plan. I look up and see that the commuters around me, surrounding me, are all men. They're all looking at me with blank faces. Some of them are absently rubbing themselves through their trousers and some of them have their penises in their hands already. And stranger number two is rubbing his own against me now, under my skirt.

[<$19,000 • Gay/lesbian • In a relationship • No]

One of my fantasies is as follows: I am a man with a 'butler' who sources willing females for me to have sex with. There are five women who are presented to me naked, lying with their legs open on a very large bed. None of them are shaved. I too am naked and have a big erection as I walk along slowly, looking at each one in turn. I feast my eyes on the juicy cunts spread out on offer. My 'butler' dictates how many I am allowed to finger, lick and fuck. He's more generous when it's my birthday. Today I can finger two, lick three and fuck one. I usually cheat a little by smelling each one, somewhat randomly, before deciding how to proceed. I take my time, looking and smelling, sometimes stroking bellies or inside thighs. I start by stroking one of the cunts, feeling its wetness, and its coming alive under my finger, rubbing the clitoris. The woman responds by opening her legs wider and pushing against my hand. I slip first one finger in, then two. I continue to pleasure her, while then licking the next pussy. I savour her honey smell and taste, exploring inside with my tongue, and alternating this with licking her clit. My other hand is stroking my cock. When they have both come I move onto another cunt, which I lick and probe with my tongue. This one has two pussies that are begging to be fingered at the same time. Who am I to refuse? I gladly pleasure them simultaneously, becoming increasingly aroused as they climax under my attentive fingers and mouth and tongue. I then penetrate one of them, sliding my cock in slowly, feeling her velvety, engorged wetness gripping me. I fuck her vigorously for a few minutes, knowing this is what she wants, until she comes, her cunt juices changing consistency. No faked climaxes here. I then withdraw and lie on my back and ask her to ride me. What joy to feel her lowering herself onto my waiting, impatient cock as another of the lucky women I have licked sits on my face. I grip her buttocks as my tongue again explores her beautiful vulva. I feel them both come again. Needless to say, I am unable to hold back much longer, and shoot my spunk in her. My 'butler' then takes his turn while I watch. He has no restrictions on how many he can pleasure.

[Bisexual/pansexual • Married/in a civil partnership • No]

It is a hot night, humid and dusky. I'm out with the girls, legs newly tanned and skirt short. Heads have been turning and I've been enjoying the attention. The bartender is flirty and I enjoy the extra shot he dishes out to me and the girls. A familiar tune comes on and we all start to dance; the air is pounding and there's sex in the heavy air. The crowd is heaving with men, playful, eager, the dance floor so packed we are barely able to move beyond dancing and moving against each other. Suddenly there's a hand on my inner thigh, reaching up and touching. Another hand is on my waist, stroking. Another comes under my top, touching the underside of my breast and feeling its way, insistently, to my nipple. I carry on dancing, rubbing myself against the anonymous man behind me. Two men at my side feel each breast; one in front has fallen to his knees in the crowded space, as though he has dropped something, but he is reaching up and touching me and it feels like power. The crowd is so dense no one can see what is happening, but I know. The man behind lifts my skirt and pushes me forward slightly, his hands feeling me and preparing me. My knickers are pulled down and then I feel it. It is rock hard, huge, deep. He fucks me while the other men watch, their hands on me, on their cocks, drinking it in. No one in the crowd can see this, no one except us. The feeling is power. It fills me. I never see their faces. I don't care. They move in and their cocks fill me in succession and all I want to do is take each one in my slick cunt.

[<$64,000 • Heterosexual • Married/in a civil partnership • Yes]

I am leaning against the bar in a dimly lit, busy pub. In the wooden bar front are several oval openings that are covered on the inside by a movable panel. Women wisely wear skirts and no knickers, standing with their crotches pressed against these panels. On the other side, hidden staff can choose which panel to open. They will secretly finger, lick, tease with vibrators, sometimes until orgasm occurs, sometimes suddenly stopping and shutting the panel. Pretending nothing is happening is glorious torture. This fantasy will work for me every time.

[Dutch • <$19,000 • Heterosexual • Single • No]

It's early evening and I'm at a party in a large manor house north of London, with friends. I've never really liked crowds, so after making the circuit, I wander off by myself. Fortunately, there are beautiful paintings and sculptures everywhere and I amuse myself by roaming the halls on the upper floors admiring them. At some point during my tour, I hear thunder in the distance, a storm heading this way. As I continue looking at the art, I find myself in what to my American eyes looks like a gallery, perhaps a ballroom when the manor house was first built. Huge, mostly empty except for the paintings on the walls.

Completing my lap around the room, I near the doorway and suddenly the lights flicker and die. I stand stock-still for a moment, wondering what just happened. I look around but see nothing in the pitch-blackness. Maybe there will be some light in the hallway, I think, so I gingerly grope my way toward the door. I find it and ease into the hallway. I stop, still not able to see anything, but I can hear faint voices from downstairs. The voices don't sound panicked, so I relax a little, realising it was probably just the storm that took out the power.

I turn and try to remember the way to the stairs, meaning to make my way back to the party, when I run up against something solid and large. I gasp as I start to fall backwards, then feel warm, strong arms around me keeping me upright. My hands are gripping the lapels of a man's jacket. I am too startled to speak or move. He doesn't move either, and we stand there in an almost embrace. He is tall and smells faintly of whiskey and a spice I can't quite identify. I suddenly feel no need to move, except maybe closer to him.

After what seems like minutes, he lowers his head toward my ear and in a husky whisper asks if I'm all right. I raise my head a little, still gripping his jacket and whisper, 'I am, are you?' Neither of us has made a move to let go of the other, his hands warm on my back. A few moments later, his arms shift and

I feel disappointment welling up inside me, but he doesn't let go, merely slides his hands closer to my waist. Then he bends his head down again and suggests we find one of the bedrooms where there might be more light. He guides me down the dark hallway until we come to a closed door. He opens it and ushers me in, closing it behind us. Still no light anywhere, not even a faint bit from the windows, nothing but darkness. Standing behind me, he leans close and says, 'Oh, too bad, no light in here either.' His voice sends shivers down my spine. 'Maybe we should just wait out the storm here?' I say.

His head brushes mine as he bends even closer, and my legs are like jelly as I feel his hands move to my hips, then his lips on my neck and he pulls me closer. I move against him and hear him growl softly. I turn to face him, wanting to taste his mouth; he obliges, kissing me softly and slowly at first, our tongues exploring each other. After a few moments he pulls back; I look up to where I assume his face was, but neither of us can see a thing. He laughs. 'Since we can't see each other, should we introduce ourselves at least?' he asks. I think for a second before answering, 'Let's not.'

I feel him lean toward me and he's kissing me again, his hands on my backside pulling me into him. I feel myself rubbing up against his hardness, my body responding in kind, my heart pounding and my breathing getting faster. I unbutton his shirt, his hands find the zip on my dress, edging it slowly downward. But he's faster than me and slips the dress off my shoulders before I can finish unbuttoning him. The dress pools at my feet and he takes off his jacket and tie. The last button is undone and I slide my hands up his chest then push the shirt off of him. I reach for his trousers, unbuttoning and unzipping. I can feel his hard cock through the fabric, aching to be freed. I push them off of him. Our mouths find each other again, licking, tasting. Our hands roaming everywhere we can reach, sliding over every inch of each other. Suddenly, I feel myself being lifted up, so I wrap my legs around him, and I can feel his cock slide in me, as if we'd practised this – many times before. I moan and he kisses me again, his tongue plunging into my mouth mirroring his cock inside me. He walks us a couple of steps and finds the bed, lowering me down slowly, never breaking contact with any part of me. We move slowly at first, then more urgently until it's too much to hold back. We both come at the same time, our bodies slick with sweat, breathing hard and fast. We lie holding each other for several minutes as our breathing returns to normal. I feel him move off of me and, for a split second, wish he was still inside me. He lies facing me, softly rubbing my hip, then laughs and asks my name. 'Why ruin the mystery?' I say. Then he leans over and kisses me. 'Perhaps,' he says and I hear the smile in his voice again. We get up from the bed and grope about for our clothes, and when we find them, I pick up my dress and slide it back on. Sighing, I say that I should get back to the party before my friends start to worry.

'Will I see you again?' he asks. 'You haven't seen me at all,' I reply.

Then I kiss him gently and slip out the door, hoping to find my way downstairs before the lights come back on.

[White American • Heterosexual • Married/in a civil partnership • No]

In my fantasy I am taken by a man I have never seen before and give myself to him with no conditions. In the hotel corridor, naked under my button-down dress and blindfolded, the door opens and I step inside. I rub myself, masturbate while he watches. He says he wants to see my finger disappearing into my cunt; that he will not touch me at all until he pushes into me when I'm coming. I really need to take a deep breath – the thought of getting hard cock in that precise moment is incredible! Letting my coming cunt contract around it while it pushes deep. I feel high. He is dangerous and I'm loving it, and I let my dress drop. I stretch my back, move my hips from side to side, sensing my own wetness leaking. I don't know where the bed is. I take a step, another and my knee touches the bedcover. I stretch my arm out, then another, and climb on it. I push my bum out, stretching like a cat. I lower my upper body, spreading my legs wide, wider, and press my head on the bed. I reach my hand under my belly and touch myself. How open my pussy is! I let my finger slide over my clit and I feel his hot breath on it, he is watching so closely. Being blindfolded, and in my own bubble, pushing my ass out to him, feeling my tight smooth ass with my other hand, sliding the finger between the cheeks until it reaches the slit of my open cunt while my other hand spreads my lips and a finger swirls on my clitoris, I am at the height of crazy uncontrollable need. All I can think of is getting his cock inside me soon. I want it now, before I come. And without sensing him behind my shaking, pushing bottom, I suddenly feel the demanding and precise push of hard flesh on my super-sensitive clit, teasing me for few seconds. And when he thrusts his cock inside my wet and hungry hole, my pulsing cunt throbs around it. I want him to fill me, not moving but just letting me suck him inside. I feel the orgasm spread around my body like a fire, making me utterly weak and powerless, a trembling mess. I have never had such an explosive orgasm. I cry, feeling something so emotional dwelling up from inside me, happiness, desperation, love even. It is just too intense. I feel his hands take my ass and pull me closer. His hold is strong: the fingers press my flesh, assuring me. He knows exactly what he's doing. We rock against each other while the waves keep coming. This is so new to me, as I usually pull away just when I start coming, often leaving the orgasm just a weak little mini thrill, never really able to make my mind leave my body. But he keeps holding me, filling me so that I keep coming and coming! I need to scream. Then he does something even more unexpected. I feel a pressure against my tight asshole, it makes my pussy and clit pop out, and his thumb slowly slides inside my asshole. The sensation is so mad, I don't know what to make of it. It is too much to bear, and at the same time I don't want it to stop. I am having another orgasm before the last one has even ebbed away, tears pouring from my eyes.

[Finnish • Bisexual/pansexual • In a relationship • Yes]

I spent the first twenty-five years of my life repressing almost everything about me in order to protect myself from a very damaging home life in which I focused on survival and nothing more. A large part of the process since then has been discovering my sexual identity. I didn't know what would (should) have been developing had my childhood and later years been normal (whatever normal means). Four or five years ago, my libido was still non-existent and sex wasn't something I even knew how to relate to. I think I was ashamed of wanting to know what I was missing, ashamed of my curiosity about my own desires. A good Indian girl doesn't think about sex and other such things ... that was my template growing up in the nineties and it fed very well into the repressed mindset I already had.

As I've worked on freeing myself from that mentality, I have tried to learn who I am as a sexual being – what do I want, who do I want, what excites me? And I have healed enough to be able to know, at least in part, what my sexual preferences might be. This is huge for me. Now, when I let sensuality dictate my thoughts, it's *my* face and *my* body I see, (short, curvy and all) and I let myself be at the centre of my desire.

I picture myself in a luxurious hotel bedroom with the ocean outside; I can hear waves crashing on the shore. I'm completely naked, lying on a large bed, a warm breeze drifting through the windows. Several extremely attractive men, all naked and really well hung, surround me on the bed, rubbing a beautifully scented oil onto my stomach and legs and feet, my back and thighs and buttocks. All over. Two of them slowly massage the oil into my breasts and stroke my nipples until they are hard. Another massages my hips; his hands slowly move inwards towards my vagina and a long finger slides between my now very wet folds: it strokes my labia and circles my clitoris really, really slowly. Then other men spread my legs very wide so I'm completely exposed and my arms are loosely tied above my head. More fingers start stroking me between my legs and more oil is rubbed along my inner thighs and some against my anus. Now slightly cold fingers slowly circle my clitoris and occasionally stroke it. As soon as I start to feel an orgasm building, the stroking fingers stop. As my body calms, they start circling and stroking again.

This cycle keeps repeating. More oiled fingers circle my vagina and clitoris and then slowly penetrate me. First one finger, then two, then three. They move in and out slowly and curve round to stroke me inside as they move. They rub against my G-spot very slightly, just enough to tease me but no more. One man licks my breasts and sucks on my nipples, the pressure slowly building. A tongue licks my clitoris and then a mouth closes over and slowly sucks on it, then the tongue pushes into me hard. It moves in and out of me faster and faster. I can feel an orgasm building. But just as I'm getting close ... again, everything stops.

The men turn me onto my stomach so I'm kneeling with my legs spread very wide, buttocks raised. They've put a raised padded seat of some kind underneath me. It has a large gap in the middle so when I lie face down on it, the area between my legs is fully accessible from beneath. Two of the men are underneath me sucking on my breasts, but this time they have small ice cubes in their mouths and occasionally slide them against my nipples. One massages more oil against my anus and very slowly introduces small anal beads. He pushes one in and then pulls it out really slowly. Then, with agonising slowness, two beads, then three ... until he's pushing the beads into me all the way and pulling them out, occasionally fast, mostly slow. Between my legs, someone puts two or three ice cubes into his mouth and pushes them into my vagina, one at a time, and then continues to push his tongue into me. The same man strokes and rubs my clitoris, using more and more pressure. Again, I'm being brought close to climax but he stops just as I'm getting really near.

Then I feel something long and hard being pushed into my vagina – one of those vibrating rabbit toys. It's slowly pulled out and pushed in again. Again, and again and again, the vibrations excite my clitoris. The anal beads are driven into me as the vibrating toy is pulled out. More fingers massage oil between my legs and then they stop; the anal beads are pushed in and left inside me. The occasional finger strokes my clitoris but apart from that, no one touches me between my legs. I feel cool, thick silk drifting across my hot skin, over my feet, my buttocks, my back, my nipples. After a couple of minutes, one of the men slides underneath me and strokes my folds with his fully erect, very large penis. He's rubbed a cooling lubricant all over his hard cock and it tingles when he strokes me with it. The silk stops gliding over my body and the anal beads start moving in and out of me again, very slowly. I feel the man underneath push his penis slowly but firmly all the way into me. He's wide and long and I'm being stretched so completely. He pulls back the hood of my clitoris so it's fully exposed, and his pubic hair strokes against it with feather-light touches as his cock pumps into me again and again.

My nipples are being sucked hard and the man behind me slaps my buttocks as he moves the anal beads in and out, faster and faster. I feel my orgasm start to build and my labia are spread wide open to expose as much of me to the air as possible. The man underneath me pounds into me harder and harder and circles his hips slightly so he's hitting my G-spot. The climax keeps building and building, and then my whole body is blazing with my orgasm. I keep coming and coming until I think I'm going to faint. Then I collapse in a heap, fully sated. I feel warm damp towels wiping me clean and I drift off to sleep.

I realise, as I finish writing this, that it's completely anonymous. The men are strangers – I don't picture my partner or anyone else I know – but I feel totally safe with them. Like I said before, I don't think I'm there yet. Or maybe I won't ever be, and maybe that's OK. My life has become all about finding out the truth of who I am, and I know this has become a defining moment in that quest. We are such fragile and complicated beings. There is so much to protect, and at times so much to protect against. That's how valuable we are. I feel very lucky to be a woman.

[Asian British • Agnostic • >$128,000 • Heterosexual • Married/ in a civil partnership • No]

The train is packed. Sweaty and tired bodies are all strewn together as we all try to get to our destinations. These people with whom I never even make eye contact, let alone strike up a conversation, flow through my mind: thinking about what their names are, fantasising what our lives would be like together.

A man steps on and sits beside me, without giving me a first or second glance. He's much older than me; greying on the sides, smile lines and a distinguished look about him. I start to feel butterflies in my stomach. Has this man noticed me at all? If our shoulders touch the next time the train brakes to a halt, would he feel the same excitement as I feel in my stomach? As the man starts reading the breaking news on his smartphone, I can't help but fantasise about him placing his hand, which is resting on the knee that keeps bumping my leg every time we go slightly faster or around a bend, in between my thighs and feeling the wetness and warmth he has created inside of me. I start worrying that my thoughts are too loud. I imagine him whispering in my ear to follow him as he takes my hand and we get off the train together and he takes me to a dark and secluded place. We finally look at each other and before I know it he's kissing me hard and pushing me passionately into the wall until I'm straddled around his hips. He kisses up and down my neck and rips my shirt to expose my breasts as his bulge, perfectly aligned between my thighs, becomes increasingly insistent. Suddenly the train stops and he proceeds to get up and exit the train, without one word or glance to me, without ever knowing what heavy petting we have just shared.

Just another stranger on a train to fall out of love with again.

[White Australian/Burmese • <$38,000 • Bisexual/pansexual • In a relationship • No]

power and
submission

'Degradation, humiliation, danger. I want all of it.'

'Lie back and think of England.' This was once a mother's standard advice to a daughter on her wedding night. Passive, meek and chaste, women were expected to close their eyes and open their legs. A century later, things have thankfully changed. And even though the most liberal-minded of mothers today may not be talking frankly to their daughters about masturbation, clitoral stimulation and the G-spot, in many countries, attitudes towards sex have been revolutionised and there is now basic sex education in schools. This progress has obviously not happened worldwide, and 'traditional' power dynamics persist in many parts of the world, extending, no doubt, into the bedroom.

As women's roles have changed at work, at home and in relationships, we've continued to make gains in agency, not only in the expression of our sexualities, but autonomy over our bodies as well. It's perhaps unsurprising, then, that in the hundreds of letters written to me, the predominant theme was that of power: domination and submission, and the sometimes fascinating dance between the two.

In some letters the domination or submission fantasy is the ultimate reversal of the everyday. One woman writes that she's a professional, a feminist, and has control over every area of her life and yet all of her fantasies centre around being dominated, degraded and humiliated by her husband. Some letters describe the inherent thrill in 'giving away the power I fought so hard to earn', while, for others, the inverse has the same effect: to take the lead with unwavering and unquestioned authority is what *generates the erotic charge. Is submitting to another's will in a fantasy a way to shut out the pressure to constantly perform and make responsible decisions in both our professional and private lives? Or does it get at deeper feelings of imposter syndrome which mean that degradation itself is, in some way, what we really deserve? Perhaps the lack of ambiguity in the sub or dom roles offer their own freedom from considerations of where we stand in a situation. Or might our fantasies of assuming authority be an embodiment of power we don't think we possess in real life? We might think of these contributions as a means of playing with and perhaps realising an increased sexual confidence. Ultimately, whatever the underlying motivation, this is what our fantasies offer us: a place where the tussle for power and control is one of pleasure rather than pain, and where women's power is harnessed and unleashed.*

I had my own experience of stepping into my sexual power in my forties when I played one of my favourite ever characters, Detective Superintendent Stella Gibson in the TV series The Fall. *Sorry to bring her up again but she did have a profound impact on me. Stella was effortlessly confident physically, intellectually and sexually. She went after what she wanted in both men and women, and it was important to me that we saw her calling the shots in the bedroom, too. I have spoken publicly about the fact that playing Stella opened up something in me in terms of sexual confidence, and also awakening a sense of femininity and sensuality. Most of us don't have the gift of a Stella Gibson to shift our own sexual narrative, but if I can get there through 'acting as if', perhaps we all have that potential within us. It's exciting to consider how we might channel our fantasies of increased power and dominion into tangible empowerment for women far and wide. And, of course, while that is a long-term project, we can at least indulge our fantasies in the meantime, a window into a potential future where our voices have unlimited power, however we choose to use it.*

•

I am what you might call a hysterical woman. I curl and uncurl my toes; I stand because I can't sit; I dream because it feels too uncomfortable to live in that feeling that comes with cancelled plans: cacoethes – 'an insatiable urge, a mania, especially for something inadvisable or harmful'. As I survey the callouses that make me half beast, it niggles between my toes. No one has ever been able to fuck this feeling out of me. But this is how I imagine it would go:

He comes in the night, strolling lightly through the stone corridors, his cloak singing a soft susurrus about him. He is tall, but not too tall. He is strong, but not indecently so. He is refined, but no aristocrat. Aristocrats don't fuck like him. He turns a corner purposefully. He has a meeting to make. In his mind, he flips through scenes before they have happened: the tearing of fabric, an urgent gasp in the stillness, the quiver of a bare leg. My bare leg. He is already hard.

He turns another corner and descends a spiral staircase. We are meeting in the dungeons. I am waiting for him, my breath stilted with anticipation. But it is not just about me; it is how he feels about me. Therein lies my desire. I can hear him now; his footsteps slow into silence as he pauses behind the door. Then he enters without permission. A fire is crackling in the grate to my left. It casts an orange glow about the room and he looks like Hades as he approaches. His face is covered; some sort of rudimentary balaclava (requested by yours truly), and his eyes shine from two black holes. They do not waver from mine. I imagine he has thought about this for weeks. Planned his movements meticulously. Tracked my own as I wandered about the castle in idle loneliness. I am in his grasp. Like he is in mine. It is debatable who is the hunter in this fantasy. I imagine the thought planted itself in his mind after I lent him some poetry. Slid it across the table one quiet evening. I imagine his clever eyes scanned the cover and his slender fingers wordlessly pocketed the small leather book, it flashing – oily in the firelight – in his motion.

I imagine him supine later that evening, the book lying belly open on his chest. I imagine for one hundred and fifty days he read it before he slept, before he washed, after he touched himself. I imagine I lay in my room with each passing minute, wondering if his lips traced the words aloud, rolling over his tongue the way his name rolled over mine.

He stands in front of me now. 'Get on your knees,' he says. I obey. The submission is in the pleasure. I can see him move in his trousers and he frees himself.

'Suck it,' he says.

He halts me just as I reach him, his fingers twisting into my hair.

'Slowly,' he says.

The detail is in the devil. Then it fills me. My throat expanding in tandem with his groan. I want it to fill every part of me; every hole, every crevice, every possible exit from one world and entrance into another subsumed, submerged, stretched asunder.

'Get up.'

His voice breaks through my reprieve. He pulls me up roughly and claims my mouth, his tongue hot and wet. A part of this desire is how much I want him. How much I've wanted him for weeks. But following his shadow around the castle is its own kind of pleasure. Being watched from afar by the thing you desire is its own kind of pleasure too. I imagine stumbling upon him gazing at a portrait of me. I imagine I can see the outline of his trousers growing larger the longer he gazes. Watching yourself be watched (I know you want me) is palpable, its own kind of pleasure. There is pleasure in waiting. He pulls my hair back now, exposing my neck. It is gently that he traces his tongue from my collarbone to my ear.

'Bend over the table,' he whispers.

I lurch towards it eagerly and it is his low chuckle that sends shivers down my spine. I bend over the table, its smooth wooden surface like velvet against my cheek. He lifts up my skirt. I am wearing hot-pink knickers – a transgression in this society where colour is considered promiscuous. He pauses, and everything is still for a moment. I squirm, impatient, and he hushes me, stroking lightly over the wet patch already showing through the fabric. 'Patience,' he murmurs. This is well deserved. Then I feel it touch me lightly over the buttocks. Leather. There's that chuckle again and a swift crack as he strikes me. I moan, and he strikes me again, and again, and again, and again, and my knees quiver. 'Please,' I gasp. I am already soaked through. He thumbs below the edge of my knickers and pulls them to the side, humming appreciatively. He forces my legs wider and spreads my lips like he owns me. I feel his tongue then, pushing deep inside me, and we exist like that for a while. And then it stops, just as I'm about to fall. He parts my lips again. I can't see what he sees, but I turn and find his eyes upon me: hungry.

'I am going to fuck you now,' he says, and he thrusts into me in one fluid motion.

I can't really say what happens next. In my head this is where the fantasy ends – everything spirals and colours merge like watercolour and it's like I'm falling down the proverbial rabbit hole. Most of my pleasure rests in the before, in the waiting. Most of my deepest desires rest in desire itself. I sometimes don't know how to say something in anything but poetry, because that's what I want – to be wanted as exquisitely as words sound resting next to one another; to be as beguiled as I am when I read a sonnet. That's what I search for – to be dominated so perfectly it is poetry.

[*British Greek Cypriot • Agnostic • <$64,000 • Bisexual/pansexual • Single • No*]

As a virgin, I have never experienced sex, but I have read and seen plenty of it around me. I realise I like to let others take the lead, and have always fantasised about being in a relationship with my boss, someone who has authority over me, someone who would tell me what to do. And though I don't actually condone it, the thought of me being married while sleeping with my boss seems all the more attractive.

I fantasise about having sex in his office, his house, wherever we could. I fantasise about him actually 'punishing' me for messing up an important project by having rough sex with me at the end of the workday, teasing me and making me beg for it. I fantasise about being tied up, whether to a desk or a chair, while I get touched in my most sensitive places. The thought of big, warm and experienced hands touching me while he tells me what to do turns me on the most.

[Black American • Christian • <$19,000 • Heterosexual • Single • No]

I am a tall, pansexual, very dynamic woman. Most men see me like a dominatrix – most women, too. But my fantasy lets me be something else. It involves a male co-worker – not someone in particular – but I imagine it is someone who knows me, meets me every day, has coffee with me. I am always fascinated thinking about how different people fuck, or come. So, yeah, it must be a male person that I meet every day. Also, I have to be this co-worker's supervisor. Now that I think of it, someone comes to mind, so I'll continue my fantasy with him.

He is not as tall as me, but very strong with a great body – he lifts weights. We are at a party at his place, lots of people. It's a hot summer night. We are drinking, dancing, laughing, flirting. People are starting to go off to different rooms to have sex. We are flirting on a couch by the pool. He casually touches my leg but immediately says sorry, as our relationship until now has been professional and friendly. At some point, we are flirting harder, I am wet and I can see from his bathing suit that he is hard. I make a joke about it and he laughs awkwardly but he looks at me with lust. I tell him that I am going to fetch something from inside.

He comes with me. Grabs me and presses me against a wall. Not kissing me, just looking. I ask him, 'Now what?' but he doesn't reply. I can feel his dick against my body. He grabs my hand and pulls me into an empty bedroom, presses me against the wall again and this time he is kissing me passionately. He grabs my ass, lifts me up and throws me onto the bed. Comes over to me and we begin kissing again. He grabs my boob and squeezes my nipple hard. I let out a little moan of pleasure and he stops kissing me, looks at me and smiles. 'I've never imagined you like this,' he says, then turns me over violently. Puts me over his knees. And spanks me. Once. The music is very loud. Twice. Checks if I'm wet – I am. Again, then again, again. As he is spanking my ass red, he leans his head down and whispers in my ear, 'You've no idea for how long I've wanted to do this.' He slaps my ass hard, grabs it. It's burning. I try to move a little bit; he spanks me harder. 'Don't wriggle!' He spanks me until I start to moan from the pain.

Suddenly he stops, puts his finger on my pussy and finds my clitoris. He then starts spanking me slowly but steadily as he rubs my clitoris. I feel my body burning, I want him to fuck me so hard. He is making me come, crying, as he spanks me harder and harder. He moves on top of me, his hard dick touches my red ass. He grabs my hair, puts his hand on my pussy. He's driving me crazy. His hand is wet from my pussy. He starts to rub my butthole slowly, it's wet, and a finger glides inside. He is whispering in my ear as he holds my hair, 'You like that?' over and over and every time I say, 'Yes.' He puts two fingers in and I move, crying out – he grabs me harder by my hair and says, 'Just tell me to stop and I'll do it.' I say, 'No, go on.' He fucks my ass with his fingers slowly. He then takes his fingers out and nudges his dick just outside my hole – without moving at first. But I start to writhe, rubbing my ass on his dick. He lets go of my hair, straightens up a little bit and starts spanking me again. Then he stops, grabs my hair again and sticks his dick into my asshole. I cry from the pain and the pleasure. He fucks my ass and I hear him moan and whisper in my ear, 'I want you to say my name.' He rubs my clitoris as he fucks me harder – I say his name many times. I am orgasming again and again as he fucks me. Then he's coming inside my ass, saying my last name – the name he calls me at work.

I think about this fantasy almost every night and I play with myself. I'm doing it even now.

[White Greek • Atheist • <$19,000 • Bisexual/pansexual • In a relationship • No]

My longest-standing fantasy, since the time I could first conceptualise sex, is being owned by an empress-like figure along with other people. She will usually command me and another person to have sex. I often imagine it happening near a waterfall in a lush forest and it always has a sort of livestock breeding aspect to it. The person I'm having sex with is sometimes eager and part of the overarching dominant sexual force. Sometimes they're nervous and coy like I am, but compelled by authority. The 'empress' treats us like pets, and is around four or five metres tall. There is a mythological goddess aspect to her, as if we're her nymphs.

[White American • Pagan • <$19,000 • Bisexual/pansexual • Cohabiting • No]

My fantasy is that I'm a lowly deckhand on a pirate ship with an all-female crew. I am straight. They are fierce women; feisty, sexy, lustful. You don't argue with them, otherwise you are stripped naked and whipped. They are all lesbians. When the ship is docked they drink rum and visit brothels. They wear loosely laced-up blouses and tight red bodices so you can see the curve of their breasts and slim trousers with brown boots.

One night, I am summoned to the captain's private quarters. It is dark, lighted by flickering candles, and I can see shapes moving rhythmically. I step inside: there are pairs of women naked, sucking and rubbing each other, groaning in ecstasy. I have butterflies in my stomach and it starts to dawn on me why I am here. I have heard whispers of these gatherings and secretly longed for and craved the feel of a soft tongue on my clit, in me, and to suck the nipples of another woman. My clit is starting to throb.

There is a group of women lying in a circle like a clock. They are flat on their backs masturbating while watching a couple fuck in the middle, like they are wrestling. Some are moaning, others are wanking furiously. The captain is sitting on a table with her legs spread wide. She is naked below her waist; she is wearing her captain's hat, her blouse and corset, but the blouse is unlaced and her full breasts are hanging out – I want to suck her nipples. She is masturbating while watching the group of women. She orders one of the other pirates to strip me naked, and then commands me to lie down in the middle of the circle. I can feel that my cheeks are flushed, and I am getting wet between my legs. The captain studies my naked body and tells the pirate what to do to me. The pirate runs her fingers lightly up and down my skin; up between my breasts, onto my neck. She holds my face and kisses me hard with her tongue in my mouth, then runs her fingers down over each nipple, down my tummy and rubs between my legs. She sucks my nipples hard. I want her so badly.

Everyone around me is fucking each other. The captain orders the pirate to straddle my mouth, so she climbs over me and starts to rub her pussy on my tongue. I want to make her come. I push my tongue flat against her clit, and poke it into her. I am so wet I feel like I need something between my legs and inside me. I want the captain to rub her pussy on me and I just want her to fuck me in any way she can; she looks so sexy sitting there, rubbing her nipples and her vagina. I don't care if she licks or sucks or grinds or fucks me with something – a candle, a bottle, anything.

The captain calls me a dirty little slut, tells me that I'm enjoying it, and pulls the pirate off me. Then she tells me she has been watching me and has been wanting to fuck me. She licks my nipples and rubs her own nipples against mine. She kisses me, holding the back of my head so I am pushed against her mouth. She lowers her head around my clit and licks and sucks, poking her tongue into me. It's ecstasy; I am groaning with pleasure, moving my hips rhythmically. But I am trying to hold off of coming, because I want to feel her clit against mine. She gets off to tease me and straddles the neck of another deckhand like me, pulls back her hair and starts rubbing her clit hard up and down her neck to get herself off. She is gasping loudly and swearing. She is looking deep into my eyes and promises me that she is going to fuck me hard next. She shudders and squirts onto the deckhand's neck. She then pushes her aside, and climbs onto me. Her clit is wet and it slides over mine. I am throbbing. I grab her and roughly pull her close, my mouth on hers. I run my hands all over her breasts, I squeeze and tug and suck her nipples sharply. I come, hard, screaming in ecstasy.

[English • Pagan • Bisexual/pansexual]

I am twenty-two years old and am told that I'm quite attractive. I play sports, swim, horse ride and keep myself fit. My fantasy is that a group of six or seven gnarly men, in their sixties, seventies and eighties, make me do things to them and with them. In my fantasy they tell me to strip for them and then they make lewd comments about my body and make me walk around as my bum is squeezed and smacked. I am told to sit on each knee as they take turns running their hands all over and inside my body. I am made to lie in the middle of them and masturbate until I orgasm. One variation is that a walking stick is used, but normally I lie there as they cheer and talk about me in very dirty language. Sometimes, I am made to stay at one of the men's houses for the weekend, and he and more of his friends take turns having sex with me for hours.

I think this fantasy comes from once being caught in the bath by a very old man and being so turned on with his eyes looking at my nakedness that it felt like he was touching me with them. He was in a complete trance for a few minutes, as I just lay there. The feeling is complete submission but a total empowerment as I am giving them something that they haven't had for years and probably never will again. It makes me feel completely sexual and is a complete release from reality ... One day, maybe.

[White English • <$19,000 • Heterosexual • In a relationship • No]

In a world where as a woman I'm told I have to control my weight, my attitude, my vulnerability, and always be on guard, I want pure release. In my everyday life, I'm a strong woman who conquers the business world. And in my average sexual encounters, I'm the dominant force. My fantasy is to not be — to forgo all control and finally give away the power I fought so hard to earn. I don't want to make decisions, I want to be told. My fantasy is to be taken care of; I want to be tied up and brought close to release over and over again. I want to be a good girl, kept in line with tiny punishments of pain that keep my body awake and my mind focused. Put me in a cage where if my posture starts to slip, spikes start to poke me. I want to be at my master's beck and call, to mewl at someone's feet begging for release.

It feels like a dirty secret that, for once, I want to be a sub. And I wish this concept didn't feel so foreign. Giving away this part of me is raw and potentially devastating. Yet I yearn for sex in which nothing can be overthought because the dynamic is set. Sex in which I'm cared for and given permission to care in return.

[Latina American • Jewish • >$128,000 • Bisexual/pansexual • In a relationship • No]

I am a feminist woman working in the legal field, who believes women should be as powerful as they want to be. In many ways, I have a great amount of control over who I am and what I do: how I spend my money, how I treat my body and the way that I dress. But I want to lose that control. And every one of my fantasies involves my boyfriend dominating me. I want him to dominate me in the way the man I lost my virginity to did. Perhaps I crave danger. A true, masculine man choking me as he fucks me. Whispering in my ear about how much of a slut I am, *his* little slut, and how proud my daddy must be knowing how much I love having a nice big dick inside of me. Slapping my ass while I'm on all fours until my cheeks are black and blue. Putting a vibrator up my pussy, waiting for him to turn it on remotely as I walk around the grocery store. Degradation, humiliation, danger. I want all of it.

[White American • Atheist • >$128,000 • Bisexual/pansexual • Cohabiting • No]

For a long while now, I've wondered what it would be like to have sex with a woman. The thought loops in my brain, therapeutic in many ways. Truthfully, it's a little frightening to put pen to paper with the fear of being judged too harshly, but here I am sharing with every ounce of courage I have. I just want to have some really wild, wild sex – uncouth in some ways – with a woman (all this consensual, of course). I like the idea of being dominated by a woman of authority, to watch her have her way with me in the mirror in front of us. I also want her to talk to me while we're going at it and she's deep inside; tell me all the dirty things she wants to do to me, rail me, fuck me brutally and shove me. I want a little bit of kink where I am restrained, with rope or leather cuffs – tied up with no control whatsoever. Nipple clamps, sexually teased, orgasm controlled. My hands bound in a very specific way behind my back, bent over or on all fours and hair pulled while she fucks me with her strap – hard and deep. The need to be overstimulated, my clit too sensitive, yet an occasional flick or using toys as part of the tease is always welcomed. Vibrating when I'm least expecting it (especially if we're out). To be spanked out of passion and not anger. I want to hurt when it's over (in a good satisfied way), not exactly the deep and dark kind but so it hurts good enough that it breaks my skin. Skin filled with scratches, love bites and marks.

I want the emotional, intimate connection we have in female friendships where we are allowed to feel comfortable enough to explore and experience each other – no room for judgement. I want to feel the gentle touch of a woman. Caressing each and every curve of my body in exploration. I want a full make-out session, getting heavier by the minute. Sometimes maybe just whispers of sweet nothings and I want all that to be done to me so I feel visible goose bumps forming on my skin but so it also has me shaking to my core, pleading for more. I want my breath to quicken, in between broken gasps and moans escaping my mouth when fingers or a tongue reach hidden places that have barely seen the light. I want her hands around my neck choking me when she gives me sloppy kisses, tells me what a good girl I've been for taking it all. A little bit of nipple play on the verge of climaxing, rolling them between her fingers while tugging on them. Slowing it down, once my nipples are hard, licking them harder and sucking till I can't take it any more, giving in to the tidal wave of pleasure coursing through my entire body. There's bound to be a string of lingering doubts about whether you can give as good as you receive. I want our naked bodies pressed together in the summer night, nipples rubbing against each other. When we pull apart, heavy breathing, lips red and bruised, I want to pull in for another and make her melt. I don't necessarily want always to be fully dominated. In fact, I like switching it up. She sometimes relinquishes control, trusting me well enough to know all the things she wants done that day, in what order and with what intensity. And I get the upper hand – a little power play in the mix. My turn to explore her body, draw circles on every inch of her skin, whisper the unspeakable things I will be doing to her. She is spread out on the desk, legs wide open, her cunt glistening with wetness, aching to be touched. I want to watch her fuck herself, one – two – three fingers in, pumping and intense eye contact between us. There is something really super-hot about it escalating so quickly, you barely have time to register what your next move is, so you go along with the flow and whatever her body responds to. My fingers deep inside her, massaging her spots till it has her moaning and squirming for more with her head thrown back. Tasting her off of my fingers. After all that, I want her to sit on my face, my tongue gently licking back and forth between her folds, my hands on her breasts, pinching them, and at the same time proceeding to suck on her clit, tipping her over the edge until she's squirting all over me and I watch her come down from a high, blissfully unaware of her surroundings. But she trusts me completely and knowing I am there for her is another turn-on, I must say.

Most importantly, sex is definitely more than just sex. Aftercare is needed. Taking the time to recover and see to each other's emotional and physical needs. Checking in with each other while we cuddle in the comfort of our bed smoking a shared joint. The euphoric feeling once it all settles in your bones. Eat and hydrate on our favourite food and drinks. An intimate scalp massage, playing with each other's hair to lull us to sleep. A personal favourite is taking turns to wash each other off in the shower, to feel more grounded, a step back into reality.

[Anglo-Indian Malaysian • <$64,000 • Gay/lesbian • Single • No]

Here is the gist of it: I'm tied to the bed. Sometimes, I have a vibrator strapped to my inner thigh and I'm forced to experience orgasm after orgasm against my will. Other times when I fantasise about it, there's nothing: I am nothing but lying in wait. The object of my desire takes on many different forms, usually modelled on whatever sexy actor or musician I'm dreaming about that week. He (it's almost always a he, despite being a queer woman myself) comes in and takes his fill of me as often as he likes. My bondage lasts all day, so he might feel the need to sate himself several times (depending on his stamina!). And I am nothing but a willing hole for him, happy to be that for him: something for him to fuck and make himself feel good. Sometimes, he gets me off in reward. Other times, he leaves me with his come leaking out of me or drying on my face, my body. Either way, I am deliriously happy, because it is *my* body, *my* cunt and *my* mouth that he is using. And he is nothing if not a generous lover. When the day is done, he is sure to run me a bath and set me free from my restraints, offering kisses and caresses to the red and inflamed skin of my wrists and ankles. He bathes me, and afterwards he praises me for my generosity and shows me as much with my very own reward – his mouth and fingers, now used to service *me*.

[White American • Non-practising Catholic • Queer • Single • No]

For a long time now, my fantasy has been about a dominant man. An affluent man with a great job who's really, really good in bed. The 'Christian Grey' fantasy. Every single boyfriend I've ever had, since I was seventeen, has been shit at sex and needed looking after in some way. They were usually skint and lacking real sexual experience.

In my fantasy, however, I'm with a man who surprises me with restaurant reservations without checking with me first. He buys me a new dress and leaves it out on the bed with a note that says 'Wear this'. I'm picked up in an expensive car, he pays for the meal of course, and then in the bedroom, I don't have to do a thing. I'm completely submissive and pleasured beyond belief. I think that's what some men miss. I don't want to be asked about dinner, and I don't want to be involved in the planning of the dates. I just want you to have enough disposable income for you to do it yourself. I think it's the freedom aspect I get off on the most. I'm not involved in any of it. A lot of the men I've slept with have been submissives, I think. They've tried to be dominant, for me, but really, they've wanted me to do it all. To perform, to make it good, to be sexy. How about *you* do it for a change?

[Heterosexual • Single • No]

I play this film in my head when I want to have an orgasm. I never see any faces. I have been chosen by a wealthy businessman to be of service to him for a year. The businessman sent his most trusted people to find the perfect-tasting pussy, the most beautiful, intense orgasm and the right-feeling vagina and asshole. I've been licked, fingered, smelled and fucked by his experts. I am right for this man because of what is uniquely me: the shape of my breasts and nipples, the flesh and strength of my thighs and ass, the scars, the smell and taste of me. It's a body that only I have. It's an honour to be selected for the businessman and I will be treated with reverence. The first week, the only thing that passes through my lips is his semen, and the only thing he eats is my pussy. I'm woken each morning by him silently pressing my thighs open so he can feast on me and then feed me his come. This forges the connection and exchange we will share for the year. The businessman chooses what I will wear to suit his mood and desire. The clothes are custom-made to his specifications. A cream silk shirt that drapes over my braless breasts and allows him to see my long, brown nipples. Black silk knickers with an opening so my vulva can be seen and touched when he wants. Sometimes he wants my pussy to be without hair. Sometimes I'll be told not to shower for a week so he can enjoy the deep smell of me. I am often on all fours under his desk, with his cock resting in my mouth, until he feels aroused and motions me to suck it.

During business meetings in his office, I stand next to him so he can easily reach my pussy, ask me to sit on his hand, play with my breasts or suck on my nipples. Sometimes he wants the smell of my pussy to be with him so he dips his finger inside me and wipes a smudge of my come under his nose to be breathed in all day. With valued business partners, he will share my precious pussy. He uses small, intricately carved mother-of-pearl spoons to gather my come for these people to taste. For a particularly high-stakes business negotiation, I am engaged to close the lucrative deal. In preparation, I am naked and completely waxed – as is to the taste of the other man. Oils have been carefully rubbed all over me so my body glistens.

The negotiation begins with me on all fours between the two men. My employer is enjoying kneading my ass cheeks as I hold the other man's balls in my mouth and gently lick them. The pressure of my employer's touch signals me to increase the intensity. I slip the cock of the other man into my mouth and begin to suck on it while my pussy is being rubbed and made wet by my boss. His fingers slip easily inside me and there is a beautiful rhythm created by his movements that I carry over to the cock I am sucking. The negotiations are going well, so my vagina and ass are offered to the guest. By now, from behind, I am red and swollen and wet. The guest presses me wide open to take me all in. There's my cloudy come all around my vulva. And my asshole is tightly closed. He wants so much to spread it open – and my employer knows this. But until the negations progress in our favour, he can only admire and smell me.

A number is reached that unlocks the possibility for the guest to put his fingers inside me. He smothers my come around my asshole – a useful tell. He tastes his fingers and increases his offer so that he can put his cock inside my pussy. My employer is enjoying watching this power play. I can tell because he's slowly rocking his cock inside my mouth. I can feel the guest getting more intense with his fucking as the negotiations heighten. He's pressing my asshole open while he fucks my pussy and I know where he wants to come: deep inside my tight asshole. My employer throws out an insane number as the intensity builds. He starts to thrust his cock deeper into my mouth. The guest takes a few more hard strokes inside my pussy, agrees to the astronomical number, receives a nod from my employer and presses my asshole wide open so he can push his cock inside, just in time for all his pent-up come to fill me. My employer lifts me onto his desk, spreads my legs open, presses his face into my pussy and begins to lick me in a way only he knows how. As I begin to orgasm, he thrusts his cock inside me to empty his beautiful load into me. I can feel the warm come of the two businessmen slowly seeping out of my pussy and asshole. The business deal is successfully closed.

[European/Australian • Jewish • <$64,000 • Bisexual/pansexual • Married/in a civil partnership • Yes]

I have a recurring sexual fantasy about a dentist. It specifically involves the dentist chair and being tied down. I don't know what it means and I'd probably be super-upset if my actual dentist tried to fuck me but do with that what you will. That's all.

[White American • Christian • <$19,000 • Bicurious • Single • No]

I am in a really fancy hotel suite. I've taken a shower, put on a fancy dress in pastel colours, like lilac or baby pink, cute underwear with transparencies and lace, light nylon tights and some gorgeous low heels. I look fantastic, and my date, a man taller than me, is in his underwear, kneeling on the floor in front of a comfy chair. I sit there and use him as my foot rest and I masturbate while looking at him; he apologises for being taller than me, and also for being horny.

After I come, I hold his face between my feet, wearing my pretty shoes. I order him to take off my dress but to not touch my underwear. I want to step on his dick with my little heels as he keeps on apologising for having an erection. He isn't allowed to look at me as I do so; if he orgasms too quickly then the date is over. But if he endures it, he's allowed to lick my pussy. And he thanks me for letting him lick me; he holds my hips as he licks my pussy as if that was the only thing he could taste, and he moans when I grind my pussy against his face. If I feel like it, I get to the penetration part. He tells me that he doesn't deserve this honour and I tell him that he's right but that I didn't have a better option. He thanks me as he puts it in. I'm still wearing my underwear, even the nylon tights because they are crotchless. He comes in my panties, which he then cleans by licking them. Afterwards, he apologises for existing, for being horny and for being a filthy loser, then I caress him and tell him he's not that bad. During the second round, he cries as he thanks me for being so kind to him and letting him be in the same room as me. He fucks me while spooning me, and he comes again in my panties, which, again, he cleans up with his tongue.

[Hispanic Venezuelan • Catholic • <$19,000 • Heterosexual • Single • No]

MY REALITY: I am a very shy female, recently diagnosed as on the autism spectrum at forty-six years of age. I've had my fair share of bad relationships in the past, have always had a hard time trusting love interests, mostly due to an abusive upbringing as a child, but also always fell quickly, intensely in love, then wasn't able to leave when it turned sour. I have abandonment issues.

I've been with my new partner for four years now, and he is my twin flame, we fit perfectly. I miss nothing with him. I have the very best sex I never could have dreamt of in the life(s) I lived before.

When I masturbate and want to come fast, I imagine being a dominant alpha male, a crime boss, who stands or sits in a soft black leather chair and gets sucked off by a blonde bimbo woman who wears full make-up, has voluminous seventies-style long hair, blue eyes, and is extraordinarily pretty, like a beauty queen. She is kneeling in front of me and eager to please. She is very submissive, loves when I give her orders, and she gets massively horny when I tell her, 'You, my fucking damn slut, I own you. Do your goddamn job!' Then she stops shortly, looks up lovingly deep into my eyes, and grabs my cock harder with her dark red manicured fingers. She has absolute trust in me to be safe, and she says devotionally, 'Yes, sir!' I slap her face, and she returns to give me the world's best blow job until I come like a hurricane. I really imagine having my orgasm with a penis instead of a clitoris. Imagining the ejaculation while I masturbate really intensifies my real orgasm.

[White Swiss • Theist/Buddhist • <$128,000 • Bisexual/ pansexual • In a relationship • No]

This is how it always happens in my mind. The key is left under the mat, as I requested earlier. She waits for me. As acquaintances in a large group of friends, you wouldn't think we even like each other, so little do we talk. Maybe we don't. Whatever we think of each other, we do this. I let myself into her house and head straight for the stairs. As I look up the sweep of the staircase she's standing at the top, in that black dress. She doesn't speak and neither do I. I brush my hand up her thigh as I draw level with her and can feel there's nothing underneath the dress. She kisses me impatiently and leans into me. I let my hands explore her body over the dress, feeling how it moves against her skin, feeling her body under the fabric, the body I'm desperate to see. We still don't speak.

I lead her through to the bedroom and turn her to face the full-length mirror. I stand behind her and run my fingers down her neck and shoulders, closely followed by my lips. I watch her relax back into me. My hands find hers and guide them to the opening at the front of the dress. She understands what I want to see. I want to see all of her. I want to see her touching herself, exactly how she likes to be touched. She looks delicious in that dress and it's a fight with myself not to strip it from her. But the image is important. It's a powerful dress, but she is not in control. She is doing my bidding and will do until I leave.

I take her to the bed and we kneel in front of each other. I kiss her passionately, pulling the dress away from her shoulders: I can't help myself. When she reaches to undo my jeans, I pull her hand away. I don't want to be touched. I want to experience the effect of her through my other senses. I want to see her, taste her, hear her and smell her. I want to observe her, to understand her physicality without clouding it with my own. I lay her down and move her fingers back to where they started, only now her clit is hot and slick and swollen. I slowly unbutton that black dress so I can run my teeth across her nipples and hear her moan in pleasure. I hold one of her hands above her head to stop her reaching to touch me. Our bodies are moving against each other in a rhythm dictated by her own fingers. Her powerful thighs moving against me, drawing me into her. I release her hand and lean back so I am kneeling between her legs. I can see every inch of her, I run my hands up her legs and pull her towards me, wrapping her legs round my waist. Her fingers are quickening as her breath gets shallower and more hurried. I can hear as her breath catches slightly in her throat; I can feel myself getting wetter each time it happens.

She goes to sit up and I push her back down on the bed – I want to see all of her. I lean down to taste her, and as I do, I hear her call out my name. I look up and hold her gaze as I feel her fingers move under my tongue. She's fixated, watching me, watching her. I gently lean on her hips and hold myself over her as I feel her start to climax. It builds fast, and as her body starts to tremble, I slide my fingers inside her. She arches her back as her orgasm bursts through her. She is magnificent. Her body slick with sweat, her cheeks flushed and her mouth wanting. I kiss her again. She is more irresistible to me now than she has ever been. I can't help myself. My resolve to remain passive has vanished. I pull her to her knees and turn her round on the bed. As my hands fall down to her waist and feel her hips push back into me, I push her forward onto her hands and knees. I don't even need to move the dress, it's risen just high enough for me to slide my fingers inside her. She moans as I do, and breathlessly calls out, 'Harder.' I know what she wants. It's her favourite. But I wait a few seconds longer, feeling how hot and wet she is on my fingers.

I quickly reach into the drawer beside the bed and take out her favourite toy. It's one of mine too if I'm honest. I fasten the straps round my legs and waist and hear her gasp as I slide the shaft inside of her. I pull her hips back against me and push deep.

Those thick thighs once again feel incredible under my touch. I finally pull the dress from her and hold her body against mine. Her head leaned back against my shoulder, I feel her tongue against mine as I kiss her. I watch her fingers move back towards her clit as I slowly move into her, deeper each time. She reaches up and snakes her hand around my neck, keeping me close behind her as she moves, once again, in her own rhythm against me. I hold her tight to me so there's no space between us. This time it's slow to build, I can see her stalling her fingers as I slide into her again – she's dragging this out on purpose, which is fine by me. I'd keep her like this all night if she could take it. She's breathing in my ear as I'm fucking her. 'Don't stop,' she whispers over and over. I have no intention of stopping. I slowly bring my hand up to her neck and gently apply pressure so she feels like she can't move. As I do this, she moans and shakes and I can feel how wet she is through my jeans. I slide my hand down to her clit and feel her dripping on my fingers.

As I fuck her, she screams out and falls to her hands in front of me. I can't help but bring my fingers to my mouth to taste her. While she lies there in front of me, I remove the straps and discard the toy. She's exhausted and I gently kiss up her back to her neck, and pull the sheet over her. I whisper to her to text me when she wants me back. And then leave.

[White British • <$19,000 • Gay/lesbian • Single • No]

The ability to seamlessly switch between perspectives that are typically considered mutually exclusive – like below/above, disabled/empowered, passive/active – are at the core of my most intimate fantasies. I was born with a severe neurodegenerative disease, making me physically weak and skinny, which fits well with prevalent notions of femininity. Only my personality never matched my appearance. As a child, I was loud, quick-witted, eager, stubborn, everything a girl was not supposed to be in the late eighties and early nineties. At school, I was the only student in a wheelchair, and there certainly wasn't anybody like me on TV from whom to draw inspiration for my teenage fantasies. I had no idea how to combine sexual initiative with my particular body, so I turned to an unlikely plot device: body swapping. In high school, I was attracted to one of my teachers. She had the authority and bodily autonomy I longed for, and I could not come up with any scenario in which I would successfully make a pass at her from my wheelchair. So, I imagined that, by some alien or magical intervention, she and I suddenly swapped bodies. In her body, I could do whatever I wanted. Climb stairs, pick up her child from kindergarten, be capable, be seductive. Using her able-bodied limbs, I could finally have sex with her, while she was occupying my disabled body. It was a way of seeing myself as active, and at least it allowed my specific body to partake in sexual activities, even if I had to imagine this body temporarily belonging to somebody else.

When I eventually got real-life sexual experience, I learned that everything I grew up believing about sex and disability was inaccurate. My intimate fantasies still revolve around the shifting of perspectives and roles, but I now know that neither requires body swapping. A powered wheelchair seat and other mechanical aids can come in handy (if you need a better angle for oral, say), but participating actively in sex doesn't depend on any one specific ability. Most of it is in the mind, so really, all it takes for me to slip into an empowered role is for my partner to recognise the possibility.

Nowadays, I still fantasise about changing dynamics, but I remain firmly situated in my own body. I might subvert a cliché – say, the hot nurse, who could be looking after me during one of my many hospital stays. She might be monitoring the ventilator I use to breathe. It might be night-time, in which case I would be stuck in bed without my wheelchair. I would clearly be the passive one in need of care, the one who can't even properly lift her own arms, whereas the nurse would be the active caregiver. But what if we changed the perspective? Not the bodies involved, rather what we expect of them? Let's say the nurse is a little insecure. Maybe she's been too self-critical in the past to fully let go with partners, but with me she can embrace her own vulnerability, since any stilted attempt at perfection is meaningless in the face of severe disability. Let's say I see her as a person with needs, not just a function, and as someone I could care for. I can't hoist her up; I can't even leave the bed unassisted, but I can tell her what to do. I can communicate my desire and ask about hers, and for me, this exchange is incredibly arousing. Putting intimacy into words. Asking for consent. Getting to know each other's bodies without assuming they work in any one specific way. I invite the nurse into my bed. I kiss her thoroughly as she bends down to meet me. I have her sit on my face and give her multiple orgasms without pausing for breath, because when on a ventilator you don't actually need to. I am the active caretaker in the scenario … and so is the nurse, because one thing I've discovered is that trying to define what counts as active versus passive, giving versus receiving, helping versus needing help, is meaningless and a bit ableist, too.

In my fantasies, I get so much out of giving pleasure to someone else. So really, I receive as much as I give, which means we are both caretakers as well as being taken care of, the nurse and me. I become empowered and strong, not in spite of being physically weak, but simply because the two states aren't mutually exclusive. Being able to fully experience both sides of the coin simultaneously is what good sex is about. It subverts difference, it overcomes the distance between me and other people, a distance mostly based on prejudice and lack of imagination. Luckily, the creative mind can overcome both.

[White Danish • Agnostic • <$38,000 • Gay/lesbian • Married/ in a civil partnership • No]

I just want to have him. To play with him, to keep him in my pocket. I want him to dominate me, to make me moan and ask for a breath. I wanna harass him, wanna see him on his knees desperately waiting for my orders. He is a perfect balance of femininity and masculinity. He is harsh, distant, individualistic, and at the same time caring, loving, tender. He denied me so many times; I have never allowed any person to do the same to me, but I just want him. He is my dearest friend and I wanna see him completely naked, and fuck him from behind. I want him to choke me. I want him to dress like a woman and have sex with him as if I was a man. I want him to dress like a man and have sex with him as if I was a man. I want him to dress like a man and have sex with me as if I was a woman. I want him to dress like a woman and have sex with me as if I was a woman. I actually am a woman but I am something different when I think about him. I am more and I am whole.

Sometimes I imagine him in the arena of the Colosseum, but instead of fighting, he is in the cage with his hands tied and tongue out. Any time a woman comes near, I shout, 'Eat her pussy until she comes.' He is exhausted, his mouth is dry, he is suffering, but he can't stop because I said so. When he has satisfied all the women for the day, I enter the arena and he has finally deserved to eat my pussy. I am the happiest I ever was. It's infinity. I love him.

[Russian • Jewish • <$19,000 • Bisexual/pansexual • No]

As a personal assistant, I am responsible for the smooth running of the office. My boss is handsome and clearly likes me ... a lot. One day, I make a terrible error and lose the company several thousand pounds. I wait to be summoned but first I go to my locker and retrieve the hold-ups I use for nights out and go to the ladies to swap my tights for them. I take off my knickers and put them in my locker with the tights. Just in time. The summons comes, I go to my boss's office and knock on the door. 'In!' he barks. As I enter, I quietly lock the door behind me. I sit down in the seat across the desk from him.

'You know what you've done. You should be fired ... but,' he says, patting his knee.

Just what I'd hoped for. I walk round and lie over his knee. He lifts my skirt and gasps to see my bare bum cheeks. He lifts his hand and spanks me. I spread my legs slightly and he spanks my pussy. I orgasm on his hand. He groans. I get up and use a tissue from the box on his desk.

'Well, that was a fair punishment,' he tells me.

[*White Scottish • Agnostic • <$38,000 • Heterosexual • Married/ in a civil partnership • No*]

This fantasy is a work in progress. Every time I return to it, I add more wants. More needs. More demands. It always starts the same way: a message to a man, laying out how I want to be pleasured. The man, who could be anyone, arrives at my door and waits until I'm ready to let him in. As instructed, he's freshly showered, smartly dressed, carries a gift. Something unexpected … anything but flowers. I watch him from the top window while I stroke my clit. He rings the doorbell and steps back, knowing I'll take my time. He looks up and catches me. We hold eye contact. He doesn't know what my hands are doing or how wet I already am. I don't say anything as I open the door. I don't offer any part of my body to welcome him in. There's no need to be nice. We both know the rules. He follows in silence, taking in how good I look. How my dress brushes the backs of my thighs. How delicate my bare feet are. He murmurs something complimentary: that he can't wait to touch me, hold me, feel me. I don't return the sentiment. I sit on the sofa and sip my glass of wine. I don't offer him a drink. He knows not to expect that. He waits with his arms folded, with that look that says: 'I'll do anything you ask of me, until I won't.'

I tell him to kneel. He does, and I tip his chin back, pushing my thumb inside his mouth and hooking his cheek to one side. I open my legs and tell him to kiss my cunt. He does, pulling my underwear to one side and sliding his tongue in. I push his head against me and grab a fistful of his hair. I ask him how it tastes, and he tells me it's perfect. Pushing him backwards, I straddle him on the floor. I grind against him, loving the friction between us. He's smiling because he thinks that it's nearly time for the switch. I slap him around the face, holding on to the power for as long as I can. He grins, and I slap him again. His body tenses. Not long now. Grabbing both my wrists, he tells me not to test him. I laugh and free myself from his grip. Reaching back, I feel how hard his cock is. He's ready. So am I. I cup his balls and squeeze them. Hard. He flinches and sits up, proving my weight holds no power over him. His breath is hot against my cheeks as he grabs the back of my neck.

Now it's his turn, he says, guiding my body backwards, trying to push me down. I resist, but knowing I want to lose. He lets me struggle for a moment and then forces me onto my back. He's straddling me now, his weight pinning me to the floor. It's the perfect role reversal, choreographed for my pleasure.

He tells me to turn over, lifting his hips to give me space to move.

But I bite my lip. 'Make me.'

He shakes his head, impressed I'm still putting up a fight.

He repeats his request, his voice is deeper now. Louder too. It's a final warning that he's about to lose control. When I giggle, he grabs me, rolls me onto my stomach and groans. He can't hold back any longer. The floor is cold against my cheek as he unbuckles his belt and lifts my dress. I pull it down again but immediately he yanks it back up.

'Enough.'

And it is, for now. He whips me with his belt. The sting of the lash better each time. He stops intermittently to check I'm OK and that the pressure is hard enough. Over and over again. He strokes my hair and tells me how good I am. Then he leans closer and whispers in my ear, 'It's a privilege to be submissive, you know.'

He's right. My body yields, and he feels it. Releasing his grip, he lets me turn over. His cheeks are flushed. He runs his hands over my body, parting my legs. He asks me how I want it. I pull him close to me, wrapping my legs around his back. We stare into each other, breathing deep. Two equals. Ready to fuck.

[NA]

exploration

'I can't get her out of my head, even when my own
husband is fucking me.'

Curiosity and play are at the heart of exploration, and though these are things that we actively nurture in children, they're often quashed when we are adults, especially when it comes to sex. It seems that fear and apprehension still exist at the intersection of curiosity, sex and sexuality. Indeed, some experts think we're living in a sex recession, where decade on decade we are seeing a steady decline in the amount of sex people are having. As an article in Esquire brilliantly put it, 'sex is like a currency that's been overprinted' – too much supply, not enough demand. When the oversupply is so boring or basic, it's no wonder women are seeking to find pleasure in unusual places.

And then there's the 'orgasm gap'. This is the gap which exists between the reported orgasm rates in men and women, and it pretty consistently demonstrates that women in heterosexual relationships have far fewer orgasms than their male counterparts. This could be why many of the letters in this section clearly show the degree to which women fantasise and climax on their own.

A survey we instigated for my drinks brand G Spot showed that a small percentage of women said they were just as likely to climax away from than with their partner – and sixty-three per cent of those women said that was because they know their body better. On the one hand, this points to a lack of communication, but also perhaps a lack of play and indeed exploration. I wonder, if you are more satisfied and have more fun with your partner, does it increase or decrease the desire to explore someone or something else entirely? If women did feel more comfortable guiding their partners in how to best give them pleasure, would the fantasy of exploring outside the relationship be less prevalent? Or would it be easier to bring the partner into that fantasy?

It is also believed that the orgasm gap is less about differences in biology or anatomy but rather because of how heterosexual men and women reach peak pleasure. Mainstream films and pornography show women having world-shaking orgasms from penetrative intercourse, cultivating the prevailing belief that this sex is 'real sex' and everything else is merely 'foreplay'. It's hard for women and their partners not to absorb this and assume that she 'should' orgasm from penetration alone. Again – it seems to me – it comes down to communication.

So, some women turn to the exploration inherent in fantasy to bridge this gap; orgasms, pleasure, release and climax abound in these letters, whether at the hands or tongues or genitals of a partner, objects or even robots. We read in this section about people embracing their desires and fearlessly charting new territory. This territory sometimes borders on the surreal, as it does when we witness one woman's vision of having sex with a second version of herself, perhaps in a bid for greater erotic self-knowledge. 'In the moment of making love to myself in this fantasy,' she says, 'everything I do is perfect.' In our imaginary worlds, there is no orgasm gap.

•

I am married to a man, but I am infatuated with a woman who lives on my street. Let's call her Edith. She moved here a little over a year ago with her wife. I don't know her that well, but she is the most beautiful human being I have ever laid eyes on. She has no idea how I feel. She is always friendly, neighbourly, but, oh, how I wish she would notice me, desire me, like I desire her. I have always known I am attracted to women, to a certain degree, but I didn't think it possible that I could feel this way about someone of the same sex. I'm not sure this is even about gender any more. It's just about her.

I have never had sex with a woman. I have only felt my own breasts, my own vagina. I want to know how another woman feels. I want to know how *she* feels. I want to know how to make love to a woman, specifically her. She could teach me everything she knows. I can't stop thinking about her, about being naked in bed with her, what I would like to do with her. I want to touch her smooth skin, kiss her soft lips, feel her breasts pressed up against mine. I want to pleasure her, make her moan, make her come. Feel her muscles contracting on my tongue, on my finger. To have the power to make her feel completely sated. For her to want me like I want her. Because I know she would have the power to bring me so much pleasure, more pleasure than I have ever experienced in my life; more pleasure than any man – no, any other person – could ever give me in my life.

I dream of our legs entwined, stimulating each other's clits. I dream of her tongue slowly teasing my entire body, finishing in between my legs, while I run my hands through her dark hair. She reaches up to caress my breasts and it tips me over the edge. I scream in ecstasy as my juices flow into her mouth. She kisses me deeply and I can taste myself on her tongue. She reaches down and puts a finger in between my legs. She fingers me slowly on the outside at first. It's still sensitive from my orgasm and dripping wet. I moan as I feel it building once again. She circles my clit with her thumb and inserts her middle finger inside me. She moves in and out, torturously slow at first. She takes one of my breasts in her mouth and gradually speeds up the pace of her finger going in and out of me. I moan louder as I feel the heat inside me rising until I explode once again, coming all over her finger. After I finish coming, she slowly slides her finger out of me and puts it in her mouth, sucking my juices off. I dream of doing all that to her as well. I want to finger her while she's fingering me. I want us to come at the same time. I want us to use vibrators on each other. I want her to use a dildo on me. I enjoy having sex with a penis. And I wouldn't want to miss out on how that feels when I am having sex with her. I cannot imagine using a dildo on her, however. I'm not sure I would enjoy it. There is only one way to find out, though, I guess! I think I would let her do anything she wanted to me, and I would do anything for her, to please her. Maybe I would use a dildo that pleasures us both at the same time, so we can come together.

Will any of this ever happen? Probably not. I can't bear seeing her so happy with her wife. I can't bear seeing her in the street, smiling and waving, making polite conversation and being unable to have her, to be with her. I know I blush every time I see her, my wild fantasies flashing through my mind. Trying to hide my embarrassment, terrified she knows I fancy her, that she can tell, that her wife can tell, that my husband can tell. I can't get her out of my head, even when my own husband is fucking me.

[White British • Agnostic • Bisexual/pansexual • Married/in a civil partnership • No]

I'm sixty-two years old and my sexual desire/fantasy is to have my husband be more open to new things and to take control. To be a little rough, toying me up, using butt plugs or, for the first time ever, having anal sex. I also fantasise about two women exploring my body, sucking on my nipples, putting their fingers deep inside me, and my husband as part of it too. Having them all have total control over my body, my pleasure. They pull and twist my nipples while they finger me deeply or fuck me hard. I want total hard passion, exploring everything, no apologies.

[White American • >$128,000 • Heterosexual • Married/in a civil partnership • Yes]

I fantasise about being in a bar somewhere in Berlin, where the female bartender invites me into a break room. It's bathed in red light. She asks me if I'd like to be a member of her sex club (but in a way it's much hotter than that). I accept, and she hands me a letter with an address and tells me to come there later that night. I arrive at a mysterious mansion. Inside, I see about ten women of all races, cis and trans, and in lingerie. They ask if I'd like to be their sex toy for the night. I consent, and then, I am. I mean, we do everything, pretty much. Vaginal penetration, anal, double penetration, oral, BDSM, whatever. I just get dommed until the morning light! Importantly, all of my partners are attentive and I feel as though I have complete trust in the women. In real life I am a cis woman who identifies as pansexual, but I never really had a chance to explore that side of me since I am in a committed relationship with a man (whom I love and intend to marry) and have been since I was eighteen. I guess in my fantasy, not only do I get to explore my sexual orientation, but I am also not expected to be experienced in sex with other genders. Because, girl, I don't know a thing about vaginas other than my own. And things like this scenario and other dreams are extremely affirming to my sexuality, even though I haven't and may never have any sexual encounters with women. Who knew a fantasy lesbian gang bang could be so empowering?

[White American • Atheist • <$128,000 • Bisexual/pansexual • In a relationship • No]

I am a young lesbian, happily dating the person I will probably marry. Why then is my most recent (and most 'effective') sexual fantasy about my male supervisor at work, who is approaching sixty? I don't know what it is — we have a very jovial, largely normal adviser–advisee relationship, and I have never before fantasised about men, or any other work colleague in the past.

The fantasy begins like this: we are at a conference together, at a hotel bar, drinking and laughing and having a good time. Gentle touches and flirty glances lead to us going to his room where we kiss ravenously and he undresses me, kissing and touching my chest. I unbutton his jeans to reveal his erect cock; I take it into my mouth and begin to give him a blow job (something I have no experience doing, having only encountered vaginas — but hey, a clitoris is just a tiny penis, right? How different can it be?). He grabs the sheets with one hand and the back of my head with the other, forcing me to take him in deeper and bringing him close to climax. He thinks oral is all he will get from me, but I move away. He looks alarmed until I pull him on top of me, and try to guide his penis inside of me. Once he's there, he hungrily thrusts into me, hard and deep, until we both come.

Other fantasies include the classic 'teacher's office' fantasy — my particular favourite is showing up for a meeting with my male teacher in a dress with no underwear on. I place his hand beneath my skirt so he can feel my nakedness for himself, and we end up having sex either with me on his lap in his desk chair, or on the desk itself.

These fantasies haven't caused any issues in the real world, and to be honest I never really think of them when I'm working with my colleague. I'm simply perplexed by their existence, and had to share.

[White • Agnostic • <$64,000 • Gay/lesbian • In a relationship • No]

There's this image of a man (though I've sworn I'll only ever see women again), whom I barely know – we saw each other less than casually years ago … And well, he's entirely behind me, inside me, his hands tangled in my hair, ripping and pulling. Mascara tears down my face, and the room smells of good pot and bad deodorant. There's still a gram of coke scattered on the table, though on the other side of him is another man, larger, taller, inside him, fucking him harder than he's fucking me. No condoms, skin to skin. Simultaneously we're all sandwiched in sweat, pain and glory – such a mess.

Still, though, there's another fantasy, one that violates a personal moral so secret, so deep down I'd never tell anyone. I'm living just outside the city; clean sheets, clean suburban home. In this image, there's a traditionally handsome man touching me softly with his rough after-work hands (like no man has). He moves my parts with care, and tells me he loves me (he means it), and together we fall asleep afterwards (I love him too). That fantasy is the one that makes me feel fucking sick. What does that say about sexuality? About me?

[White American • Non-conventional but raised Southern Baptist • <$64,000 • Bisexual/pansexual • Single • No]

I am a young adult and I've had sexual relationships with men and women. My relationship with sex and gender is confusing and continues to be a journey with a changing destination. Before, I had dreams of what I wanted during sex, what I saw myself doing or what I desired someone to do to me, but that changed a few months ago after I had sex for the first time. It was with a man and it was utterly disappointing. In the build-up I was aroused, but we went two rounds and both times I felt nothing. No one's surprised that he came both times.

Now, I moved on and have found a lovely woman that I've been talking to for a while. It's nothing sexual yet, but I obviously hope it will turn that way. And this is where my confusion with gender sets in. Sex with women is nothing strange to me; I've seen it plenty of times – though I know porn can be fake, I still think I'd find my way while doing it. But my idea of having sex with a woman is me penetrating them with a penis. I don't have a penis, and I don't mean a dildo or a strap-on. I've tried masturbating to the idea of having sex with a woman with a strap-on, but that never works like me imagining a penis attached to my body. In my fantasies I see myself with a penis, though nothing else is vivid – for instance, I'm not sure if I'm a man in this scenario or still have the rest of my female body – but I am having sex with a woman and I'm fucking her, quite roughly, with my penis.

This has made me wonder if I might be transgender, but I've come to the realisation that in my magical horny world, I simply want to fuck women passionately, as a woman, with *my* imaginary penis. I'll just make sure I do a much better job at pleasing the woman than my first time with that bloke.

[*White Dutch* • *Atheist* • *<$19,000* • *Bisexual/pansexual* • *Single* • *No*]

Sometimes I still think of this sweet guy I once dated. He was French, young and blond; he had a feminine face and the way he smiled was capable of melting mountains. It was a long time ago and we lost touch – I don't know if he's dating anyone, or if he's married, what job he does and no clue where he lives either. With time I can imagine him less and less; his accent and his delicate facial features, once so dear to me, are fading from my memory and now blend together into some less-defined blondness, and what I remember of him has mutated into a sense of tenderness.

When we dated, he had little sexual experience and I was glad to be his teacher. There is one thing I always wanted to do with him but never dared to ask, and which, after all these years, I still daydream about. It all started during carnival. I was putting some red lipstick on my lips, and looking in the mirror, I saw behind my reflection that my French date was looking at me. 'You don't need lipstick to look nice,' he said. I smiled: guys always need to compliment the girl without make-up. But at that moment, I thought I would very much like to put some lipstick on his lips. Feel free to imagine what happened next, but what I am more interested in is what *did not* happen; or, let's say, in what happened in my fantasy.

This is how it goes: with some background music and a glass of red wine, I open my closet in order to try on different outfits, for me and my date. Of course, I only own girls' clothes, but, being carnival, he plays along. What about a skirt? Or those high heels? I try to convince him to choose from my selection of clothes, from the dark sparkly to the semaphore yellow. Something hot, something short, something girly. Please. Once he chooses his outfit, I also wear mine: a strap-on dildo I had bought long before and that rested unused and sad. I then make love to my French boy from a different angle, Oh yes, I push him onto the bed, pull his skirt up ... I imagine entering him, with the same tenderness he had entered me before, I imagine whispering French words of love, caressing his white silky skin. I could spend hours petting his blond hair, his thin neck, his juicy asshole. Most of all, I would like to do to him what guys have done to me, like some sort of reciprocation, experiencing the other side of it.

[White • Atheist • <$19,000 • Heterosexual • In a relationship • No]

My most guarded and secret sexual fantasy is only that because to tell it to anyone would seem vain. It is not vain, however; it is simply all-encompassing. This is why I am so thrilled to finally say it out loud: my biggest and most secret sexual fantasy is *me*. I had a very vivid lucid dream a few years back. I was at a formal business gathering in a hotel. Drinks were flowing and people were looking to hook up. In this dream, I went back to my hotel room alone. I had given up on finding someone to bring back with me, which suits me in the real world and added to the lucidity. As I was getting ready for bed, there was a knock on the door. I answered it and standing in front of me was *me*. It wasn't a twin, it wasn't a clone. It was *me*. But on the other side of the door, I was also 'me'. And I let me in, and I let me sit down on the bed with me. I charmed myself rather nicely, as you'd expect. I kissed my mouth, I kissed my neck. I touched me in all the right places with all the right vigour and lust. At this point there is no differentiating which one of me was at the door and which in the room previously. I am both me, but I am only one person. I am feeling every single thing I do to me as both the giver and the receiver. I tear my clothes off of me and discover that I have a beautiful and strongly erect penis, but I also have a vagina that is yearning. Each of us has one or the other but it interchanges. I'm shoving myself flat onto the bed like a hungry animal and I'm devouring every scrap. Sucking the bones dry. I can thrust myself into me, and I can feel what it's like to be inside of me while also enjoying what I already know. The sighs and moans are strange and eerie, as they're sounds I've heard only in my own head before this. I make love to myself so gently and passionately, and I fuck myself so hard and choke myself and I pull my hair. I'm screaming for more; I'm saying 'go slower'; I'm asking myself to speed up ... but I don't need to. I am just doing and it is *exactly* what I want. I'm up against a wall. I'm on the floor, I have rug burn. I've turned myself over and I'm in me so deep and so hard from behind. It hurts but it's amazing. It's beyond amazing, it's supernatural. When I come, I don't even know what to do. It's magical to orgasm two times at the same time.

I tried to figure this dream out; I tried to make it a metaphor. But it is exactly what it is. *To be able to be exactly who you are and receive exactly what you want.* To feel what you're giving and not just receiving. In the moment of making love to myself in this fantasy, everything I do is perfect. When I am making love to my partner in reality, I do to him what I would want done to me. When he is pleased by it, I have envy. I want to know what it feels like for him. I want to know if the emotions that are wrapped around our lovemaking or our fucking are the same or not. It doesn't matter. I just want the knowledge, the feeling. My ultimate secret fantasy is to be both them and me.

[White American • Pagan/Buddhist • <$128,000 • Bisexual/ pansexual • In a relationship • No]

I discovered, later in life than was ideal, that I am bisexual, leaning more toward having an attraction to women. I married a man before I allowed myself to learn more deeply about my own sexuality. I was also a virgin when we started dating and have only been truly intimate with this one man. I get turned on more by the female form than I do the male, I masturbate to fantasies of being with a woman, and I prefer WLW (women loving women) porn to heterosexual fare. I am thankful for my rich inner world so I can fantasise about something I may never have the chance to experience in real life.

However, the difficulty is that at times it makes me sad or depressed to accept the possibility of not being intimate with another woman as long as I live. Often, this realisation hits me while having intercourse with my husband. For example, if he sucks on my tits, I try to imagine a woman doing that to me instead. Sometimes my brain cooperates, allowing me to experience pleasure with the fantasy and the act itself in tandem. But other times, it completely takes me out of the moment and erotic headspace. To expand on the example, I get so bothered that I may not ever be able to suck on another woman's tits. I want very badly to know what it feels like to take a woman's nipple into my mouth or to dip my tongue into her sex. I want to run my hands across soft curves while my head is nestled between her legs and give another woman sexual pleasure. I am not that adventurous in the bedroom, but I think I would be if I was with a woman. When my husband expressed a desire to include ass play, I went along reluctantly, letting him lick me there and fuck me in the ass with his fingers. I found it to be very stimulating and I enjoy participating in this act when I am the receiver. I have no desire to reciprocate for my husband and he understands, happy that I enjoy it when he does it to me. Shortly after introducing this into our sex play, I had the same sudden realisation, that a woman will most likely never pleasure me in this way. Then came another disheartening epiphany. If given the chance, I would definitely engage in consensual anal sex (giving or receiving) with another woman using toys, but the thought of doing that with a man just doesn't do it for me. I think I would be more demonstrative with my love and affection were my partner a woman. I might have a whole different attitude regarding sex if I hadn't committed myself to a man early on in life. Most of my fantasies involve an alternate persona where I am free to explore sexual desires with whomever I so choose. And I strongly believe I would choose women over men most of the time if given that freedom. This leads to a rather bleak outlook on my romantic and sexual future.

I confess, I do fantasise about divorcing my husband in order to feel that kind of freedom; but it remains that: a fantasy. I also fantasise about being a widow. I don't actually wish to lose my spouse, but sometimes I think about a future where he dies and I am still relatively young enough or physically able to engage in sexual activity. I dream about what it would be like to openly flirt with a woman or take one out on a date, and I often fantasise about hooking up with other women. What would it be like to have a sexy one-night stand? I want to experience so many aspects of a lesbian relationship, but I may never be in the position to do so. As a result, my fantasies are embedded with a particular longing, a yearning for a path I did not know existed when I was younger. The act of fantasising is complicated and bittersweet for me, but it's also a part of my identity. I'd much rather know these things about myself than not. It allows me to understand myself on a deeper and more compassionate level, which is important as I find myself living a life I wouldn't choose for me now.

[Italian and Portuguese American • Atheist (raised Catholic) • <$128,000 • Bisexual/pansexual • Married/in a civil partnership • Yes]

more, more, more

'I am a pleasure station! They take turns with me, teasing themselves in my mouth.'

As British music-hall artist Marie Lloyd once sang, 'A little of what you fancy does you good.' Well, never mind a little of what you fancy – it seems that many women around the world are aroused by the idea of having a lot.

We received so many fantasies about threesomes, moresomes and thensomes – with every imaginable combination of gender identities – that they outnumbered every other theme in this project. Maybe this interest in multiple partners springs from a want to reinvigorate sex in a long-term partnership, to bring back some of the insatiable excitement of a new lover? Or maybe it's an expression of longing to play outside the confines of a relationship, without jealousy or repercussions – to experiment and discover? Or perhaps it simply comes from a desire for a sexual experience that is just more: more bodies, more desire, more sensation, more gratification?

While filming The Crown, in which I played Prime Minister Margaret Thatcher, I was sent a piece of erotic fanfiction involving Mrs T, Labour leader Neil Kinnock and Soviet President Mikhail Gorbachev. I was understandably shocked that anyone might find that fantastical scenario even remotely stimulating. But, as with other group-sex fanfic that I've been alerted to over the years, particularly involving my character Agent Scully paired with Agent Mulder and FBI Assistant Director Walter Skinner, I know that there is a living, breathing universe out there where lifetimes are devoted to crafting *these surprising, if not bewildering, fantasies and sharing them on public forums. Along with everything in life, 'to each their own'.*

For some women, their multiples fantasies involve people they know – their partner and a friend, a series of ex-lovers who know their body and how to turn them on, even the neighbours. For others, the joy of a multiples fantasy is that it can be set anywhere, with anyone – in a monastery, pleasuring the monks, or a special kind of commune where each man has three wives. For some, the sex is an end in itself, and yet for others it's part of a polyamorous lifestyle, like one woman who says, 'I want multiple husbands who all know and like each other. I want them to have other wives. No one owns anyone.'

Humans are one of the few species for whom monogamy is the norm. This can inevitably change and dampen sexual desire over time – familiarity and repetition can foster intimacy, tenderness and care, but does not always cultivate eroticism, which thrives on the new and the unexpected. The injection of novelty offered by group sex is ripe for fantasy and has a long-established history. Here we find an insatiable hunger and an endless pursuit of orgasm. While modern life can feel like a trundling hamster wheel of progress towards more success or money or status, the pleasure in these fantasies is the goal itself. As one woman explains, 'When I'm in a boring meeting or sometimes on the bus, I disappear into my dirty fantasy life and I'm a million miles away, getting endlessly fucked.' There's something liberating and pure in the idea of pleasure for pleasure's sake and these fantasies represent a rare opportunity to be fully and intensely present in that moment of exquisite pleasure.

•

On the surface, I am a frumpy fifty-year-old with a weight problem. I live an ordinary life and have the typical interests and hobbies of a middle-aged American woman. My actual sex life mirrors the sad trajectory of many long-term marriages. Sex is rare, and when it does occur, it's as if my husband has completely forgotten what foreplay is. He is impotent and the medications help little, so I am left hungry for penetration. The thought that I'll probably never have great sex again depresses me so much I retreat from reality. People would probably be shocked if they ever got a glimpse of my vivid fantasy life, and that thought makes me smile.

In my mind, I don't bemoan my ageing, fuller-figured self; instead, I am young and curvy, full breasts and long legs. Beautiful and sexy. My alter ego feels no shame, and doesn't hide her libido or desires from anyone. No act or partner is off limits. Through her I get my sexual hunger sated, indulging in amazing sex with handsome men whose sole desire is to please me. In my mind, I get penetrated all the time, and in some very small way it makes up for what I lack in reality.

My most basic fantasy is to be gang-banged by a group of men at a sex party – all the hard cock I can handle, with no refractory period and certainly no impotence. I'm in a big, beautiful house where men and women wander around, some barely clothed, some nude, all wearing masks. The lights are low and the air smells of incense and female arousal. Moans and sighs of pleasure become background music. I'm wearing a robe over a baby doll and black lingerie, lace and satin clinging to my curves as my long hair falls over my shoulder. The men in this scenario are large, over six feet tall and beefy, all with giant cocks. They circle me as I lie on a bed, their soft hands touching my hair, my breasts, my pussy. One man fingers me while I suck on another's cock; someone else goes down on me while I jerk off a couple of the other men. A handsome man leans over and strokes my face, then kisses me, his tongue sensually dancing with mine. Finally, when I'm so aroused I can barely stand it, one of the men pulls my legs apart and slowly pushes his giant cock into me. He thrusts into me languorously at first and I quiver at the feeling of him inside of me, hitting me in all the right places. The other men caress my body and kiss me everywhere, taking turns to present their cock to me to suck, and every few minutes I pleasure someone new. The man fucking me moans in his arousal and tells me how great my pussy feels as he grabs my thighs and pulls me closer, trying to get even deeper. His moans become louder and he jerks, coming in me in long, hot streams. I can feel his warm come slip out of my pussy and down to my ass. After he catches his breath, he pulls out of me and moves away.

Another man takes his place and pushes my legs apart and slides into me. He also has a huge cock but it feels different than the man before him, and I revel in the unique sensations of his hardness caressing the bumps and grooves of my pussy. He slams into me so hard I inch up the bed, and he has to drag me back down by my thighs. I want to come, I tell him, and he puts his thumb on my clit and rubs in circles. The sound of my moaning drowns out his grunts of exertion. I'm climbing the mountain to that beautiful place of light and peace and ecstasy, and he climbs with me. I reach the peak and I scream, convulsing all over his cock as I fly through my orgasm. Just as I am beginning to come down, he pulls his cock out of my pussy and strokes himself, coming in thick white ropes all over my tits.

Once he catches his breath he steps aside and lets another man in between my legs, and after this man comes into me there is another waiting in line, and another, and another, and the fucking starts all over again. The line of men is long and I never have to wait more than a minute to be filled up by another huge cock.

These men and their beautiful cocks come to me when I use my vibrator and when I'm attempting sex with my husband, but they make frequent appearances at other times, too. When I'm in a boring meeting or sometimes on the bus, I disappear into my dirty fantasy life and I'm a million miles away, getting endlessly fucked. So, the next time you see a plain, large, middle-aged woman, don't be so quick to overlook them, or to assume they have average, boring lives. Maybe they do, but their internal selves might be as wild and free as mine is, full of lust and sweaty bodies and endless fantasies.

[White American • Witch • >$128,000 • Heterosexual • Married/ in a civil partnership • No]

My fantasy is no secret. I want multiple husbands who all know and like each other. I want them to have other wives. No one owns anyone. No one is obligated to stay. Everyone feels safe enough to be honest. Friendship is the first commitment; sexual affection grows from that mutual respect. Sharing affection instead of hoarding it makes for more love to go around for everyone. Sexual energy can be the most healing.

[Other/Mixed • Church of Art American • <$19,000 • Polyamorous • In a relationship • Yes]

As one of many in a sea of transgender women, I've realised that hormone therapy has a huge effect on our sex drives. Basically, forcing our bodies to go through puberty twice and all that comes with that. Personally, during hormone therapy I had something of a second awakening with fantasy and drive. I went from being just OK with the thought of men to indulgently full of desire for their sexual equipment and the wonderful fluids they produce. Most of my dreams revolved around multiple guys at once! Sometimes up to SEVEN. SEVEN! It was not something I was used to ... going from a mild-mannered person to someone who liked to end up looking like a cinnamon roll on the regular, with extra frosting.

[White American • Agnostic • <$19,000 • Bisexual/pansexual • In a relationship • No]

In my fantasy I am living a glamorous lifestyle similar to my great-grandmother's. I am a sexually explorative New York flapper in the 1930s. A renowned singer at a speakeasy, I break all the rules that are expected of me as a woman during this era. I am unabashed and confident and complicated and enigmatic. I exude sensuality within my ruby-velvet garments and glistening pearls, and my sultry voice mesmerises the patrons who arrive for me and only me. I finish my set and an attractive couple offers to buy me a drink, but I get my drinks on the house, so I order us each a round. The man is friendly, easy-going and collected, with dark slicked-back hair and a cool sense of style. The woman is shy and intimidated. Perhaps she is awestruck. Perhaps she wonders if she is enough for me. I take the couple up the spiral staircase to my apartment, where I assure them that clothing in the heated pool is optional.

We soak together and enjoy each other's company and the woman admits that she has always imagined kissing me. She says this as our legs wrap together, and I oblige her with the press of my lips. The man is overjoyed by the direction of the night, but he is not allowed to touch until I say so. He pours us some more wine and the wife and I slow-dance under moody lighting to Ella Fitzgerald, still naked and dripping wet from the pool. The man watches with deep, desperate breaths and I reach out to him and he comes from behind his wife and sways with us both. The wife is hardly interested in him, as her attention is solely on me. We then move into the living room where my collection of dramatic art, masks and sculptures surround a grand fireplace. We cuddle under blankets and warm ourselves by the flames and the man asks if he can rub my back. I agree to it, and as he does so, the woman begins to kiss and lick my breasts. She bites softly and sucks to the point where I can feel it in my groin. She kisses me down the centre of my stomach and to my vulva, while the man takes hold of my breasts and continues massaging. I feel his cock rub against me, but he hasn't earned me yet. I tell him to go down on his wife, and he does for me to watch. The woman's eyes are never taken off me, even as she comes. She says she wants only me and so I climb on top of her and let her eat my pussy while I suck on the man, and just as he is on the brink of orgasm, he throws me onto the couch and pulls my legs over his shoulders. He enters me easily and pounds me until I'm practically exploding from the power of his cock. As he comes, I can hear him. His release is like music. The woman is in tears from the beauty of having watched her spouse fuck me without constraint. Impressed and shaking with pleasure, I cover myself in a luxurious robe and offer crackers and dips to balance out the wine. The couple is gracious and they wish to stay but I cannot commit to their love. Certainly, I may see them again, but there are other fans that seek my affections, and until someone gives me reason to return the love, I remain free and elusive, sharing my king-sized bed only with the many feline friends that take up its space.

[Russian-Jewish American • Pagan • Bisexual/pansexual • Single • No]

I'm in my twenties and still a virgin, which I'm quite ashamed of sometimes, as it feels like everyone has had their first time in their teens. But this doesn't mean I'm not a sexual being, nor that I've never had an orgasm. While I'm pleasuring myself, I have sexual fantasies – sometimes about women, sometimes men, sometimes even both. So, for now my sex life basically consists of fantasies. I'm incredibly insecure about my looks, and don't feel comfortable in my own skin at all. To say I hate my body might be a bit too harsh, but it's certainly close to it. I guess that's exactly the reason why I haven't had sex yet: if I can't love my own body and feel comfortable with it, how will I be able to believe that someone else finds it attractive or even sexually appealing?

My fantasies are always about meeting someone who really likes me with all my scars, my cellulitis, stretch marks, loose skin ... someone who makes me feel attractive and sexy, allowing me to forget about my insecurities. In one, I meet up with this lovely couple at a gorgeous, cosy hotel; I don't know them in my everyday life and we've never met before, but we all want to try something new sexually.

When I see them for the first time, I am stunned. They're around my age, maybe slightly older. He is tall, sporty, but not too muscular, with greenish-brown eyes and short dark blond hair. She is a small, slim, but very feminine, with big blue eyes and long blonde hair. One of those couples you can't help notice when they pass by on the street. But I immediately feel more drawn to the woman because of her self-confidence, elegance and femininity. After a drink at the hotel bar to loosen up a bit, we go up to our room, the three of us squeezed into this narrow lift ... I feel my excitement build as I take a closer look at the woman; her elegant nose, her oh-so-kissable lips. And she smells heavenly. I realise that I am staring at her and draw back a little, but she smiles at me, leans in and kisses me, her soft lips, softly pressed against mine, tasting so wonderfully sweet and slightly like the drink she has just had. I could stay like this forever, exploring each other's mouths, but the lift pings and we walk down the corridor to our room. My legs a little wobbly and my heart beating wildly, it feels like miles. As soon as we close the door, the woman and I kiss more passionately, forgetting everything around us for a moment, even that the man is watching us. But we've planned something different for tonight. They've always fantasised about being watched by someone while having sex. And I've fantasised about watching a couple.

There's a huge king-sized bed, an armchair and a desk in the corner of the room. I sit in the armchair, and as I watch them kiss passionately and slowly undress each other on the bed, I can't help but touch under my clothes. She is on top, taking control, which really turns me on. As they're about to reach their climax, my heart pounds faster and faster in arousal and excitement.

Afterwards, I switch places with him. I look at her, naked and out of breath, literally glowing. So self-confident and content with her own body. She smiles at me, happy and seductive, then she kisses me. Passionately. She undresses me and I want to stay here forever, in this room, in this moment, kissing this beautiful woman. I don't even notice that the man is sitting in the armchair, watching us. She takes a moment to look at my naked form with a soft smile on her face and desire in her eyes. Then she pulls me against her and we keep kissing, pressing our bodies closer, touching each other, exploring each other's bodies with our hands and mouths, both fully letting go, quickly learning what the other likes, pushing exactly the right buttons. Teasing each other, pleasuring each other and having wonderful orgasms together. I feel completely comfortable with myself and am able to fully let go of all my self-consciousness. I am confident and able to ask for what I need and want, sexually and in every other way, too. My body feels like it's on fire and I feel like I could fly.

[White German • Agnostic • <$19,000 • Bisexual/pansexual • Single • No]

My fantasy is that the neighbours have invited me over with my husband. Not our actual neighbours but fantasy neighbours. We have a drink and some nibbles, then they say they want to have a threesome with me. I am game and I start kissing the wife while the husband watches us. My husband seems to have left, so I get things going with the wife and then the husband. I have never had a threesome and doubt I ever will, as I'm in my seventies. But, well, a fantasy is something else.

[White Australian • Jewish • >$128,000 • Heterosexual • Married/ in a civil partnership • Yes]

Growing up, I was sexually attracted to guys but never did much because I lived in a strict household. But that gave me time to think about how I want to have sex. I want my man to wake me up and touch my body slowly and tell me how beautiful I am. Kiss my neck while grinding on me. But at the same time, I crave to kiss a girl and just scissor her while my man jerks himself off. I want a threesome but I don't want to share my man's dick. I want to eat a girl out while I get eaten out. I want her to touch me in all places while his dick is only inside me. I want to scissor her with a vibrator on me so I can come while he finishes on the side. I want to be shared but I don't want to share.

[Hispanic Mexican • Heterosexual • In a relationship • No]

One of my favourite fantasies that gets me going every time is where I'm seduced by a lesbian couple. Many, many years ago a very attractive, very sexy couple hit on me on the dance floor. I was at a fancy party and I ended up separated from my boyfriend, dancing with strangers, and before I knew it these two gorgeous women started moving with me. It was clear what their intentions were and if I had been braver, more adventurous, not in a relationship? Who knows, perhaps I would have followed them home. Ever since then, whether I'm alone touching myself or my partner's head is between my legs, I've fantasised about what would have happened if I had.

It starts with us still on the dance floor surrounded by sweaty bodies, all moving to a sexy beat. One of the women is behind me, her whole body pressed against mine and her hot breath in my ear. The other has her firm rear grinding against my crotch to the rhythm. Two sets of hands grasp my hips and we move as one.

The brunette whispers something about getting out of there and grabs my hand. I reach for the blonde and we weave our way towards the exit and the truck they have parked outside. We slide into the long front seat and as one of them drives, they each have a hand on me somewhere, stroking, teasing. I'm nervous. I'm excited. It's incredibly hot. I've left my boyfriend behind! Inside their apartment, we make small talk. The brunette brings me a drink and when I take it she leans in and presses her soft lips to mine. We stand in the middle of the living room and we kiss, gently at first, almost chaste, and then deeper and faster and hotter, our tongues exploring the insides of each other's mouths, our hands starting to explore each other's curves. I notice that jazz music has started to play, the lights have been dimmed, and then … we are joined by the blonde. She takes the drink from my hand and presses herself against me from behind, her hands on my hips, her lips on the back of my neck, her fingers making their way slowly over my ass, gently inching up my skirt and finding their way into my panties. I am soaking wet.

She moans into my ear as she slides a finger deep inside me and lowers herself to the ground, burying her face in my ass. I can feel her hot breath through my summer dress, her finger moving in and out as I move my hips against it. Meanwhile the brunette, who has been feasting on my neck, moves down to my breasts, her tongue lapping at my nipples. My knees are getting weak. Together they slide my panties down to the floor as they lower me to my knees. The blonde positions herself underneath me and my pussy onto her mouth. I am so close to coming. Her hot soft tongue gently licks and pulses inside my lips. The brunette moves between my breasts, my neck and my mouth, her teeth gently biting here and there as I squirm and moan and writhe and cum deeper than I ever have before in my life.

[White American • None • Pansexual • In a relationship • Yes]

In my fantasy I have been taken in by the monks at an isolated hermitage. As the only female, I become the happy participant in many activities, some ordered by an older monk who appears to be the leader. I have housekeeping tasks in the ancient stone building we all share. I want all the members (pun intended) to be happy and they all care about my happiness as well. I carry out daily 'duties', which include fellating any monks who pass me in the hallway, waking them all up in the morning by lowering myself onto their faces or their eager cocks. I make sure there is variety in our daily 'activities', and at the end of the day I regale the abbot with stories of what I've done. He masturbates me as I tell him and my orgasm is the culmination of a very enjoyable fantasy.

[White Canadian • Atheist • <$64,000 • Heterosexual • In a relationship • No]

My fantasy was sparked on a girls' holiday, a bachelorette to be exact. At the airport we were all exhilarated by the idea that on this holiday 'anything goes' as, technically, this was the last time the bride-to-be could legally have fun, with no repercussions. As we boarded the plane to Marrakech, already two glasses of wine down, I knew it'd be a holiday to remember. I think it was on the fourth day that the fun started to dry up. We had done everything – drunk our bodyweight in alcohol, skinny-dipped in the sea, shared our craziest sex stories, drunk-texted old flings – and now we were truly out of ideas on how to 'one-up ourselves'. I'm not sure who suggested it, but the idea circulated that we should go to a sex party, 'Just to look of course', 'Just out of curiosity of course'. So, we did our research and found the red-light district equivalent in Marrakech. When we got there, there was a feeling of scandal and tension in the air. It was exciting, but unfamiliar. And none of us girls knew how to act. We sat frozen, only allowing our eyes to scan the room. We were all secretly waiting for someone else to initiate something. But nobody did. In the private rooms, mostly men were pleasuring each other. And even the women who were there seemed to be roped into pleasuring another man. So we went home. But I couldn't stop thinking about what I saw in those rooms. I found myself wishing that things had gone differently. That there had been more women. That somebody met you at the door to welcome the nervous first-timer. That they had provided sterilised toys for those who were more self-conscious. Until, finally, I had created a full-blown fantasy in my head.

Ever since that night, I have had a recurring fantasy of starting my own bachelorette sex-dungeon business. All the details have been ironed out. I'd advertise the event as explicitly for groups, ensuring I had their age and consent. I'd welcome the guests as normal, offer everyone a drink and maybe a feather boa for good spirits. Then I'd direct the bride into a private room and tell her that her bridal party had arranged a massage for her. I'd massage her and, eventually, ask if she'd like me to go further. I'd come equipped with toys and make sure she got her happy ending. Afterwards, each person in the bridal party would have a chance to experience my private room, while the others continued to drink and party in the main hall. It would be a night of total ecstasy for everyone, celebrating women's pleasure. You may ask, how is this a fantasy for me? Well, I'd find great satisfaction in pleasuring each woman and, quite frankly, getting paid to do it. If any of the women wanted to go a step further without the toys, I'd happily oblige.

[Black Caribbean British • Agnostic • <$64,000 • Heterosexual • Single • No]

It was years before I allowed myself any fantasies during sex. Decades, really. In all those years, I felt that any fantasy made me disloyal to the man I was with, so I consciously silenced even the first hint of my imagination going somewhere else. In my sixties, however, a consistent fantasy began to emerge. Interestingly, it always includes my husband, plus two other men who are dear friends and who I know really value me. In this fantasy, all three are touching and loving me everywhere, all at once: with tongues, penises, hands, bodies, they caress and penetrate and stimulate and delight me. The collective impact of their joyous collaboration: I feel utterly beautiful, utterly adored. Without guilt! As a child, I felt unloved and unworthy; as an adult, I have grappled with those self-esteem challenges. At seventy-two, I am unapologetically enlivened and enriched by three wonderful men, loving me everywhere, enthusiastically, deliciously, simultaneously.

[White American • Jewish • >$128,000 • Heterosexual • Married/ in a civil partnership • Yes]

The fantasy starts how I like it to end: I'm in bed, asleep, with all the best of my past lovers – the respectful ones, the hot ones, the ones who know what I like and how to give it to me. They are all beautiful, beautiful men. There are maybe fifteen of them, maybe more. I'm woken up by one of them stroking my knickers over my pussy, his fingers pulling my underwear to one side and opening my lips to feel my wetness. I can see in the half-light how he is excited by me, by my body, my presence. He slips his fingers into me and touches himself at the same time. Slowly the others wake up little by little, like lions sleepily watching the prey that they know they will have later for dinner, and they are enjoying the show. One brings a length of rope and ties my legs together up to my knees, slowly, respectfully. I can see his hardness, how he takes pleasure from this moment. I feel the rope tight around my skin as another feasts on me, on my pussy, on my arse. He quenches his thirst with me.

I rub my fingers over my lips, showing them how plump they are and how I will be wanting their cocks on them later. I am bound, but *I* am the one in control. *I* am the object of desire and I own it. I love it, as I love all of these men who are pleasuring themselves by pleasuring me. I have orchestrated this situation and I have chosen these men for this journey. I am now on my front, legs still tied, and I am rubbing a cock on the outside of my lips, a nice hard one, a beautiful cock. I rub it over my lips and face. I enjoy this so much, I lick around, bring my lips full over the gland, back and forth, every so often I envelop the whole thing with my mouth and start again. The man is moaning and arching with pleasure. I tease him with my lips. I take him to the brink and back. Others watch, hands around their cocks.

I feel hands caressing me, a spank, fingers inside my now very wet pussy, inside my arse. Another spank. My thighs glisten with my wetness. A third spank, and a fourth. The binding ropes are removed and I am showered in caresses and kisses over the sore bumps where they pinched my flesh. The sensation of the rope marks makes me even hornier. Kisses on my neck, bites that immobilise me, like a kitten, fingers squeezing my already hard nipples, cocks left and right waiting for me, wanting me. Fingers inside me, outside of me, massaging me. I am in the centre of pleasure; I am reduced – or elevated – to pure feeling, to joy. Slowly we fuck, sometimes in my pussy, sometimes in my arse, sometimes both. The men take great pleasure in watching each other make love to me. They take pleasure from my pleasure. I come, again and again, rising up on waves of my and their excitement. I come with their cocks, their fingers, their weight on me – sometimes just looking at them makes me come. Sometimes I place myself at the top of the bed and I touch myself and I watch them, watching me, wanting me. Someone fingers me harder and my pussy squirts; I love this sensation of *lâcher prise* – this moment when I am not in control. I am, for a short instant, totally at the mercy of the others. It is again pure joy to be desired, touched, caressed by all these gorgeous men. There is a lot of laughter, a lot of tenderness. We are playing at lovers. They don't all come – that's not the end goal – but one might ejaculate on my arse, his cock rubbing between my cheeks until he does. One might come while watching me fucking. Another may come on my breasts or in my mouth, but not everyone, as this journey lasts for hours, the whole day even. There are breaks while we sleep, and then I am woken up again, to fuck. And then at the end, we all go back to sleep together, curled up like a basket of kittens, exhausted and full of oxytocin.

[White French • <$19,000 • Heterosexual • Married/in a civil partnership • Yes]

My ultimate fantasy is something that I truly hope comes to fruition someday. I imagine it happening while I am on vacation with my husband of ten years. We are staying at a beach resort with incredible views of the ocean. We are at a swim-up bar, drinking and talking to other guests, and strike up a conversation with a woman who is there on her own. She is beautifully curvaceous and has a beautiful ass. We have a great time talking to her, she and I getting up to dance together when there are songs that we just can't help dancing to. My husband watches on as this woman and I are caressing each other, swaying our hips in perfect sync. After dancing particularly passionately to one song, we are hot and our hair is a mess. We both go to move the other's hair out of her face. The fact that we are so in tune makes us smile and slightly giggly. We look into each other's eyes for a long moment. Our breath quickens and subconsciously we lick our lips. She still has a hand on my waist as her chest rises and falls rapidly and she bites her lip.

I look over to my husband who smiles. I look back at her and can hardly catch my breath. I run my hand slowly from her stomach to her waist and, maintaining eye contact, gently pull her closer. Just enough of a nudge to let her know where I would love this to go, but not so much that she couldn't break the tension and connection that can be felt surrounding us. Her mouth falls slightly open and her lips are plump and glistening. She gasps when we make full contact. Breasts to breasts and pelvis to pelvis. I keep my hand on her waist and with my free hand I stroke the side of her face while gently nudging her head closer to me so that our lips touch. It is so gentle and sensual. I pull back ever so slightly so that I can see her face. I want to make sure that she wants what I want. She looks at me with such heat that I feel like I am going to melt under her gaze. She brings her hand up to my face to caress my cheek and then reaches round to grab onto my hair. She grasps it firmly at the base of my neck and pulls so that my face tilts up to hers. She is making sure that I am aware she has taken control. When she pulls my hair a little tighter to gauge my reaction, I gasp and rub my body against hers. Then she kisses me. Our tongues are entwined and I am writhing against her as she pulls harder and gives me the sweetest bit of bite. I know that if she put her mouth to my other, lower lips, I would feel pure bliss. Suddenly she pulls back and stares into my eyes. There is hunger there, and deep in my groin, my core tightens. I know that look of pure desire in her eyes is for me. We turn to my husband, who is breathing heavily – our actions have excited him. She asks if we should go to her room or ours. I glance at my husband to make sure that he is right there with us and he says, 'Ours.'

As we make our way inside, she keeps her body close to mine, as if she can't stand to lose the contact. Waiting for the elevator, she kisses me passionately, slowly running her hands over my waist and the sides of my breasts, as if she is trying to memorise my body by touch. Thankfully the elevator is empty apart from us, and as soon as the door closes, the woman and I lock eyes. I smile at her mischievously and we both turn our gaze on my husband. We then step slowly toward him, like hungry animals stealthily approaching our prey. I grab his ass, pull him to me, grinding my pelvis against him to see how excited he is. I can read his body easily and know that he is in the moment and happy with what is unfolding. I gently pull the woman in too, and she presses herself against his hip and allows her breasts to brush his side, tentatively at first, testing the waters. Then I give her a deliciously naughty smile and pull her in more closely so she knows that everything is OK with me. She grinds herself against him harder and starts to moan deeply. Her breath quickens. I know that she is close to getting herself off, so I pull her back toward me. I want her orgasm to be explosive, not over in an instant in an elevator.

We quickly burst into our suite. I push my husband against the wall and lick his throat. I feel him as he quivers from the sensation. She is still a little unsure of touching my husband since she doesn't want to upset me, so I give her a salacious look and guide her closer so that her pelvis is pressed against his cock and her breasts against his chest. I push myself against her and put my hand on her lower back as I whisper to her, 'Want to have some fun with us?' She nods her head frantically as I run my fingers over her, as if I have all the time in the world to caress her entire body. I want her to know that I will take the time it takes to make it an amazing experience for all of us.

I keep rubbing myself against her back and ass, gyrating slowly. At the same time, I caress my husband to spur him on. He starts to kiss her and I run my hands over her upper body. I increase the pressure as I run one hand up under her shirt, the other inside her bra to fondle her breast. My husband takes her mouth with a kiss. Her nipples are very sensitive and I can feel how turned on she is. I take one of her nipples and roll it gently between my index finger and thumb. She breaks the kiss and arches her back, moaning loudly. I start to kiss and suck the side of her neck, while grabbing my husband's hip and pulling him into our embrace, making sure that we are all connected. We both grind against her in total sync, making her moan and whimper. I slide my hand down into her knickers; she is soaking wet and she hisses as I lightly brush over her clit before putting two fingers inside her. I curl my fingers each time I slowly thrust in, so that I hit her G-spot each time. She is whimpering because she really wants to get off but it just isn't enough. I thrust a few more times to really get her on the edge of coming, but stop right before she can get her release. I pull my fingers out of her cunt and she cries out in protest. My fingers are drenched with her juices and I hold them out to my husband who slowly sucks her honey from my fingers with a deep and dominating moan. I sit on the bed. He has her pressed against the wall right inside the door. They're gyrating against each other, mouths open, can't catch their breath. They're climbing to their peaks while I watch, the woman going wild with the need to orgasm. She presses herself against him and he reaches between her legs to rub her clit, bringing her to the brink of climax. He looks to me, but I shake my head, no, so he stops. She whimpers in frustration, then he leads her over to the bed and gently places her next to me, and I start caressing her and rubbing myself against her. I give him a subtle nod. He kisses her before stepping back, then we both watch in lust as my husband strips off his clothing. Once he is naked, she and I lock eyes and we slowly strip for him. Then she is eating my pussy like it is the juiciest and tastiest peach on earth. I scream out in ecstasy at the pleasure she is giving me. Meanwhile, my husband is riding her from behind. I quickly come, her magic tongue devouring me. Now she can't help succumbing to him. She moves up my body and is now on top of me, face-to-face. She is looking into my eyes as he rides her from behind. I keep caressing her and holding her shoulders against his thrusts. She cries out loud that it is so deep and that it feels too good. She places her pelvis close to mine, kissing me as he drives into her from behind, one hand on the back of my neck, trying to hold on to anything against this onslaught of pleasure. Her other hand is against my crotch, her fingers thrusting into me as the force of my husband pushes against us, so that, easily, she makes me come for her again.

She looks at me with desperation clear in her eyes. She too wants to come, so badly. I bite her neck and hold her shoulders to force him deeper into her, then she grips both of my hips with desperation as she comes harder than she ever has before. My husband then reaches his climax and we all just lie there together for a moment, like a sexy sandwich.

[Asian and White American • Agnostic/pagan • >$128,000 • Bisexual/pansexual • Married/in a civil partnership • No]

In my fantasy, I am a new woman arriving in a community in which there are certain rules and guidelines to living out one's sexuality and partnership. Newcomers are inducted through a period of initiation under instruction from the male leader (the most powerful man in the community), which involves extensive sexual opening and tantric practices, after which there is a ritual in which every man in the community makes love to me, as a kind of welcoming and sealing of the web of belonging I am now part of. For this second phase, I must wear some kind of accessory that marks me out as belonging to every man who wishes to have sex with me. As the newest member of the community, I am aware of all the attention I receive and of the men lusting after me. And also, the tension in my budding new friendships with the other women around me, feeling their jealousy, knowing that their husbands come and visit me during the day. In the final initiation phase, I am 'given' to a man to be one of his three female partners. The rest of my fantasy plays out in the intense lust and emotional charge of not being the 'only' one and having to wait for my 'turn'. What arouses me the most is the fantasy that I am the 'middle' wife, and that there is an older wife who is jealous of me, and an even younger wife who is pregnant and whom I am jealous of, and yet extremely titillated by the sexual appetite and fecundity she shares with the man I am devoted to.

[White German • <$38,000 • Straightish • In a relationship • No]

Not long after we met, my husband and I were watching porn together. There was one video I never forgot, of a man sharing his wife with a friend. This is my fantasy. I'm on my knees, tied to the kitchen island. My husband and a mutual friend are in the kitchen. They're keen amateur cooks and have been talking about cooking a roast together for a while now. I wait patiently as they discuss how they'll work together. The friend comes to me and smiles, pulls my top down and exposes my breasts, tugging them roughly from the bra cups and arranging them so they stand out. He gently plucks, pinches, rolls and teases my nipples for a few minutes while he and my husband finish their discussion. His groin is at my eye level and I can see he's getting excited. It gives me a thrill. Then he slaps both of my breasts smartly a few times, so they bounce together, pops a grape into my mouth and turns to do some chopping. Presently my husband comes over and blindfolds me. He pulls himself free from his trousers, lays his penis against my chin and I obediently open my mouth. He hardens and swells in my mouth, holding my ponytail in his hand. He keeps my head steady as he glides in and out of my mouth for a moment, then pulls away. I am rewarded with a sip of wine. I am a pleasure station! They take turns with me, teasing themselves in my mouth. They intermittently fondle, squeeze and slap my breasts, giving me pleasure and titillating gentle pain so I become a horny desperate mess. Once the final food preparations are done and the roast is in the oven, they release me and I am led to the sitting room. They position me on my hands and knees on a wide footstool. They know how hot they've made me. My husband stands before me and slips his penis into my mouth again. Our friend watches from the shadows, stroking himself. He approaches me and slides his penis into me from behind. They slap me, stroke me, tease me and fuck me until I feel like I will come without assistance. Then our friend slowly circles my clit with his fingers as he fucks me, my husband pinches my nipples hard as he pounds into my mouth and I come; it's intense and it leaves me shaking as they use me until they too have come. Only then do they remove my blindfold. Afterwards, we cuddle together on the sofa to wait for dinner. I feel wonderfully used, but heady and powerful. To be wanted and treated as I want to be treated by two men I respect is (I believe) liberating. I drowse, satisfied, and listen to them planning dessert ...

[Irish • Heterosexual • Married/in a civil partnership • Yes]

I used to think it was weird to like anal sex. Only women who wanted to please men did it. How could they enjoy it? But then I started dating someone with whom I was ridiculously sexually compatible. We experimented with new things and I began to understand why some people like it. I enjoyed the feeling of him inside me with a sex toy as well. And now I crave two cocks. I imagine it. Sometimes I dream about it.

My fantasy is to have two men inside me at once, front and back. I'm sure there is a word for it, though I don't know what it is. I have seen it in porn. Threesomes, as often pictured by men, are of two women at their service. But I want two men to fill me up. Double penetration. I don't know who these men would be. I'm not sure it really matters. Perhaps this means I am guilty of objectifying them – for the sole pleasures of their penises – like women so often are for their breasts, bums, bodies. But I do know that these men are kind and patient and they ask me whether it feels OK; checking in throughout, listening for my audible cues. Breathing, body succumbing to pleasure. Slow, gradual building. Never sudden movements, no surprises. They enjoy it too, of course. That matters tremendously to me. We are all enjoying it, no fake noises, no performances. It would begin with a massage and body oil. Yoni and lingam massages, everyone touching everyone. Silky shafts, glossy vulva. So relaxed and ready that our faces are glazed with want. Our appetites longing to taste and enjoy each other, almost with desperation. A deep thirst being quenched. We move on to tongues and lips and licks. Enjoying sucking and lapping, in distinguishing bodies. Everything builds, everything bulges, everyone is holding out for the delicious finale, but really, truly, savouring the entrée.

In my fantasy I am filled. Full up. Full-filled. I hold my small vibrator, buzzing it on my clit. It is all I've wanted for so long. We all come at the same time. A physical and mental release so powerful it lasts for the rest of my life. Residual euphoria. I am no longer insatiable, I am full.

[White British • Atheist • <$128,000 • Heterosexual • Cohabiting • No]

the watchers and the watched

'Thinking about them watching me while I pleasure myself drives me wild.'

O ne of many undeniable shifts that have occurred since the publication of Nancy Friday's My Secret Garden in *1973* is the role that social media now plays in our lives. We have become, in a very short space of time, a society divided into the watchers and the watched. Some of us want the eyes of the world on us at all times, performing, showing off, exposing ourselves and the mundane and the extraordinary in our own lives. This pseudo intimacy and its quick-fix dopamine hits in the form of likes and follows makes Peeping Toms of us all as we become obsessive voyeurs of other people's lives. And at the click of a button, any of us with access to the internet can also watch any flavour of pornography, if we so wish. It's no wonder that our sexual imagination and fantasies are fuelled by an innumerable assortment of these accumulated images. But in our personal, private movie reel, we are simultaneously both the audience and the actor, the subject and the object. Fantasies, like dreams, don't need to conform to rigid rules of realistic casting: we can shift between roles depending on our desires; we can imagine ourselves as highly irresistible sexual agents. And we can play at being on both sides of the lens – being watched and watching others.

As someone who is watched for a living, I have a complicated relationship with privacy. When I'm playing a role, I am completely at ease with being watched, whereas in my personal life, I feel self-conscious and constantly aware of the gaze of others. Some days I wear it lightly and on others it feels like a burden. If I had

*my druthers, I would move about the world invisibly. And indeed,
at the very heart of all my own fantasies, I am the watcher, not the
watched. Or sometimes I switch between watcher and participant,
but I am most definitely the director. The privacy of my own mind
is the one place where I am truly in control of when, how or even
whether I am seen. It's pretty clear from these letters that I am
not alone, not only in my desire to be in control and have a say in
my desires but, perhaps most importantly, to be seen through the
female gaze.*

•

I fantasise about watching my husband fuck another woman. It's not a fantasy I would ever share with him, because I don't know how I would feel if it actually happened. But it's always the same. We were on a cruise about fourteen years ago and, on an excursion off the ship, there was a beautiful woman with us who was flirting with him. Later, I saw her on the ship and she was wearing a form-fitting white dress. I fantasise that I bring her back to our cabin and tell my husband that I've brought him a surprise. The woman unzips her dress and strips totally nude and I tell him he can do whatever he wants with her. Then she tells my husband that she's been dreaming of fucking him all day and he tells her he wants to see what she's been imagining. I watch her suck his cock and then ride him until he finishes inside her. This is my go-to fantasy while he's eating me out and I always orgasm from the thought of it.

[White/Native American • Christian • >$128,000 • Heterosexual • Married/in a civil partnership • Yes]

My deepest sexual fantasy is being used as a study tool for medical students. I am in the centre of a large stage, with around thirty medical students of both genders surrounding me. They are allowed to look and touch wherever they like, all for the purposes of studying the female body. They are all looking at my vagina, looking and learning about the different areas and gently touching it, poking around. I reach orgasm with them all watching professionally and taking notes.

[Asian British • <$38,000 • Bisexual/pansexual • Single • No]

As a woman who is nearing thirty, married and child-free, I have my fair share of relationship problems. I'm overweight and my husband isn't attracted to me sexually. Most of the time sex for me is trying to please him with oral and then when he is done he leaves the room and I finish myself off with my vibrator. As stimulation, I fantasise that I am pegging my husband and then making him watch as his best friend fucks me in front of him. I think because I want sex more than him, it puts me into a more masculine state of mind and I want him to submit to me. By that same token, I also want to be the feminine figure that's lusted after, pushed up against a wall and ravaged by someone strong and caring.

[White American • <$19,000 • Bisexual/pansexual • Married/in a civil partnership • No]

As a working wife and mother of three small boys, sex for me is a fast and perfunctory act behind closed doors in a dimly lit bedroom with the muffled cry of 'Mommy!' being called out in the adjacent room. We're in the midst of work obligations, doctor appointments, sports practices, diaper changes, nose-wiping, dinner-making and dishwashing. My nightly reprieve after bedtime is to fold laundry, a task I used to despise, but almost relish now because it's finally quiet in my house. On cold winter nights I've contemplated crawling into the dryer because it's warm and peaceful in there. Sometimes if I try, among the cacophony of thoughts and the logistics of fulfilling everyone's needs, I catch a glimpse of my voice; myself. I think about what I want, what I *need*. The thought of being sick and bedridden enters my mind, seeming like a nice reprieve, but the whole ship would go down without me to steer it.

So, where does sex come in? The honest answer is, it doesn't. Currently, I am not getting any kind of satisfaction out of it whatsoever. It's become one-sided and obligatory, literally an item on my to-do list. We are physically so close – he's literally inside me – but I'm emotionally removed and mentally miles away. And when it's quick, I'm grateful.

However, I do revel in the lush grasses in my mind and can pleasure myself in a matter of minutes by fantasising about a couple engaged in raw, hungry sex. He fits the cliché of tall, dark and handsome. He's long, lean and muscular. Six-pack, nice pecs, defined biceps, but not overly so, athletic in a natural sort of way. She is petite and her body is sun-kissed. His is too, but not overly tanned. They're realistically beautiful. I'd say she resembles me, but better and toned in all the right places with bigger, perkier breasts. She lacks the stretch marks and squishy midsection of a mother of three. It's unclear if I'm her or if I'm merely a voyeur watching this attractive couple fuck. I haven't really worked out the point of view in my mind because it's irrelevant to the fantasy. If I'm her, I enjoy watching me with this Adonis. There's something about this couple that makes their love forbidden. There's an 'I want you, but I can't have you' vibe that permeates the moment. They're star-crossed lovers and sex is their forbidden fruit. This intensifies the moment, making the mood driven and urgent. Sometimes he's on top, sometimes she is. Regardless, there's one action that gets me off. At the most pivotal moment, their foreheads touch, they pull back slightly and, despite the reflex to ride out their orgasms internally, he forces her to keep her eyes open. Their bodies are connected; now the intensity of their gaze unites their souls. They climax nearly simultaneously. Sweat-glistened and satiated, whoever is on top slumps onto their partner and buries their head in the crevice of his or her neck. I realise it sounds like something from a damn romance novel, but it's their desperate, burning, emotional connection that arouses me the most.

I'm sure my husband would love to know this secret that gets me off, but I'd rather keep it to myself.

[Bisexual/pansexual • Married/in a civil partnership • Yes]

I fantasise that one of my executive directors calls me into his office. I'm wearing a white blouse, pencil skirt, no panties. The office has glass walls and anyone who walks past can see inside. He has me face his desk while he walks behind me. Slowly unzipping my skirt while undoing his trousers. Pulling his hard penis out. Sliding it inside my wet pussy because he knows I want it bad. Fucking me non-stop until I drip come down my legs.

[Hispanic American • <$128,000 • Heterosexual • In a relationship • Yes]

I am sixty years old and the fantasy I've had since quite a young age is as follows: I have been taken to the cinema by my boyfriend. We are in the back row and when the film begins we start to kiss and fondle each other. My boyfriend is touching me everywhere and undressing me. I don't object because I am enjoying it. Before I realise it, he has removed most of my clothing when, suddenly, there is an interval in the film and the house lights come up. At this point, I realise that the rest of the audience in the cinema is made up solely of men. I feel slightly panicked until my boyfriend takes me by the hand and leads me up on to the stage of the cinema. I am standing naked in front of all these men. My boyfriend declares that he is going to 'display' me so that everyone can see every intimate part of me and then he is going to invite the audience to have a closer look at me. He states that they can look but cannot touch. He also tells me that he is going to choose several of the men to stand over me and pleasure themselves until they ejaculate over me and that they can choose where they want to ejaculate. I am scared but excited at the same time, as I feel vulnerable being naked but protected by my boyfriend, who is clearly excited about showing off his beautiful girlfriend.

That's about where it ends because by this point I will have come to orgasm and feel satiated. I have never told anyone about this fantasy. It has always been my secret and the place I go to when I want to orgasm. I have never orgasmed through sex as I have never been able to completely let go with someone else, not even my husband. I have been with him for forty years this month but we have not had sex for about twelve years due to impotence problems brought about by diabetes. I haven't used my fantasy for a while as I have started to experience orgasms during sleep (not frequently but frequently enough!) that I find absolutely sensational.

[White English • Protestant • <$38,000 • Heterosexual • Married/ in a civil partnership • Yes]

I love my wife, but she seems to have lost her libido. So, what I think about during sex is actually what I think about during masturbation. Not even my wife is aware of my sexual fantasies, though she is aware that I fancy some men. My sexual fantasies almost exclusively feature myself partnered up with guys. Maybe the fantasies seem less like cheating if I'm with a man instead of a woman. Maybe I'm into how ostentatiously lustful men generally are compared to women. Whatever it is, in my fantasies I'm rarely with a woman, despite being more attracted to women both physically and mentally in real life.

Over time, my fantasies have evolved into being more extreme sexual encounters in order to be able to get turned on, things I wouldn't necessarily be into in reality. I've got to imagine being ogled, having multiple spectators, having multiple partners, exhibitionism, voyeurism and some light submission. A typical session for me starts with meeting up with a man I know and trust. I'm dressed a bit too provocatively for general public consumption, but just the right amount to drop some jaws. My nipples being visible through my clothing is a favourite. (#freethenipple and all that, but I do get wildly turned on by women's breasts, so I imagine it's just as exciting for straight men.)

Sometimes my gentleman takes me to a party dressed like this so that he can observe others ogling me. Sometimes he invites friends and strangers to our location to see their reactions to me. Unsuspecting pizza-delivery guys are a fun one. Let's go with that one. When the delivery guy arrives, I'm instructed to answer the door. There's an unspoken agreement between my gentleman and me that I'll do whatever he says. This is where the submission part comes in. Delivery Guy is surprised at my visible nipples and what is usually a short skirt with pretty panties and a garter belt underneath. I've been instructed to drop the payment and to do a revealing bend-over to retrieve it – another treat for Delivery Guy. When he's properly enticed, my gentleman comes to the door to strike a deal. Would Delivery Guy prefer cash for a tip or a little something more interesting? He, of course, chooses what (at first) is a look at my breasts. The next time he delivers (yes, this is a long play), the tip he chooses is to touch my breasts with his hands. The next delivery, he chooses to touch my breasts with his mouth. (Ignore how often this means we have pizza – and even though this would happen over several weeks, it's all in rapid succession in my mind.) The tip progresses to his being allowed to look at my pussy, then touching my pussy. It culminates with him being able to have me suck his dick as a tip while my gentleman watches. Why doesn't it culminate with him fucking me? Because only my man gets that privilege.

Sometimes I invent scenarios that anger my man so that I need to be punished with a spanking, which is always a spectator sport. I'm only spanked when others are there to watch, and sometimes they are asked to participate. When it's finally time for my gentleman to fuck me, this happens with several spectators. It's the final treat for everyone and it's my final delight as well. By the time I get to this point in my imagination, I am fully turned on and ready to come.

[*White American* • *<$38,000* • *Bisexual/pansexual* • *Married/in a civil partnership* • *No*]

My fantasies usually unfold as if I am the man in the situation, which as a woman is probably quite strange. My husband has a very low sex drive. If I make the effort to turn him on, when he's not tired or busy, it works. But to my shame, I find I can't be bothered a lot of the time. It's easier and more pleasurable to simply fantasise and get myself off. I masturbate several times a week. I find it very erotic to imagine how a man feels as he's about to come. I also love the idea of being watched and of watching others.

My current go-to fantasy is about a man whose wife is performing in a live sex show on a small stage. I imagine that I am the husband, watching both her onstage and also the audience. The seats are starting to fill up with couples and individuals, all quite giddy about the performance they're going to see. My wife pops her head round the curtain and gives me a small wave. Her eyes are shining and I can tell she's already feeling horny at the thought of having sex in front of an audience.

I turn my attention to a couple in the front row. The man is already sporting a large bulge in his tight trousers and the woman has noticed it; she raises her eyebrows and runs a fingernail down the length of his hard-on. He smiles, slightly bashfully, and leans in to kiss her passionately. She arches her body towards him and he briefly fondles one of her breasts. The sight makes my cock pulse in my jeans. I notice that another man behind them is also watching the couple and is lightly stroking his cock through his trousers.

The lights come up onstage and my wife enters in a maid's uniform. Her magnificent tits spill out over the top of her blouse, and her black skirt is so short that if she bends over she will expose her pussy. I hope she's not wearing any panties. She reaches up with her feather duster so you can see the tops of her stockings. Then she moves round the bed and bends down to 'dust' the skirting board. My heart skips a beat and my cock hardens as I see the slick of her pussy lips, shining in the stage lights. She's wet already. I lick my lips and my cock throbs in my jeans, but I resist touching myself yet.

A young man joins her onstage but she seems not to notice, carrying on with her 'dusting'. He's incredibly good-looking, muscular in all the right places and wearing a tight pair of trousers that outline his thick member. There's a gasp from the tense-looking lady on my left – her eyes are glued to the young man onstage and her handbag is now rammed into her groin. Another woman in the row behind reaches inside her blouse to finger her breasts, pulling at the nipples and biting her lip. My cock pulses knowing that all these people are being turned on by my wife.

Onstage, the young man clears his throat and my wife leaps up, pretending to be horrified, trying to pull her skirt down. He smirks at her and tells her to come over to him. She does, looking apprehensive. He runs a hand over her tits, round her bottom and down her thigh and then slowly up the inside of her legs and the gasp she gives tells me he's just reached her pussy. Her eyes widen and he tells her how naughty she is, coming to work with no panties on. Did she want to get caught? She says 'No', but her chest is heaving and I can see her nipples pushing against the front of her uniform. She's incredibly turned on. My cock is aching now and I rub it through my jeans. I know if I get it out now and start properly touching myself I'll come far too quickly, so I force myself to take my hand away.

The young man tells my wife to bend over the bed, she complies and I can see her juices shining on her swollen pussy lips. He pushes his hardening cock against her leg. She trembles slightly. He reaches round and cups her breast, and she whimpers. His cock is fully erect now. He tells her he can see how turned on she is and he smacks her bare bottom with his hand. She cries out and I hear a moan come from the woman with the handbag.

She is wriggling on her chair now. All the men in the audience have visible erections; most are stroking them through their trousers, but a couple have already got their cocks out. The man in the front row guides his partner's hand to his and she strokes it, while he reaches under her skirt; I see her legs spread slightly and her head snaps back as he finds her clit.

On the stage the young man roughly pulls my wife up and turns her round to face him. Would she like to feel his cock like the naughty girl she is? he asks her. She nods vigorously and reaches down to feel him through his trousers, her hands trembling as he reaches forward to kiss her passionately. A flash of jealousy passes through me, but I'm too turned on for it to last. He unzips her uniform so it falls to a puddle at her feet. She's standing naked in front of him except for her high heels and stockings. The sight of her makes me groan and I can't contain myself any longer. I pull out my throbbing cock and start to stroke it. I lock eyes with the lady in the front row; she winks at me and turns her attention back to the stage.

My wife is stripping the young man now, running her hands over his taut body. His cock leaps up as she pulls it free of his trousers. She drops to her knees and runs her tongue over it. A man in the audience groans and I hear the frantic sounds of his cock being worked hard, then he comes, semen spurting from the tip of his thrusting member. The lady with the handbag rocks rhythmically back and forth with her legs parted, jamming her bag into her crotch, rubbing herself on it and moaning as she watches my wife licking and sucking on the young man's throbbing cock.

Pumping my own cock and wishing it was the one in my wife's mouth, I feel my orgasm starting to build, so I slow it down. I don't want to come too soon. They've moved onto the bed and my wife has her legs spread wide, so the young man can go down on her. She's whimpering and flexing her hips up towards his face, and when he finally drives his tongue down onto her clit, she groans and grabs the sheets tight in her fists. She's writhing and I can tell she's close to orgasm. I groan and my cock swells in my hand. It's pure agony as it sways and throbs in front of me. The couple in the front row have changed positions; she lifts her skirt and lowers herself onto his hard cock, until it's fully inside her. He guides her hips backwards and forwards, and plays with her clit while she fucks him.

The young man onstage stops sucking and nibbling my wife's clit, lies down and instructs her to ride him. She's given up any pretence that she shouldn't be doing this and I watch her eagerly lower herself onto his huge hard penis, inch by inch, wishing fervently that it was my aching cock she was taking deep inside her. He plays with her engorged nipples. She throws her head back with pleasure and starts to match his thrusting hips with her own movements, rubbing herself against him. I can't help myself, I take my cock back in my hand. I can hear the lady with the handbag moaning loudly now. She's going to come. The couple in the front row are fucking harder. He's grabbing at her tits and she's rubbing her clit, faster and faster. The young man flips my wife over and starts pounding his cock into her, she's got her legs round his waist, telling him to fuck her harder, to make her come. I am pounding at my cock frantically now, close to ejaculation. I hear the sounds of the audience, the groans and sighs as their orgasms hit. My wife suddenly shrieks that she's coming, she looks directly at me, her head rolls back, her eyes scrunch shut, her mouth opens and I can't hold back any longer. The orgasm bursts from me as wave after wave of pleasure hits.

[White/Indian British • Church of England (lapsed) • <$64,000 • Heterosexual • Married/in a civil partnership • Yes]

When we speak of fantasies, we think of something that we could never tell our loved ones and especially our partners. In this case, bisexuality and orgies are what get me hot, breathless and excited. Not only that, but the idea that men leave their toxic masculinity at the door and withhold nothing, not even their deep moans and groans for the world – or the neighbours – to hear. I fantasise that I am watching men fuck each other while I sit back and revel in their sounds and fight over power. I want to be called upon, making sure I can command their attention without touching them. I want to be hunted. Eaten, made to feel worshipped, all while watching a group of men worship each other in ways I cannot compete with. There is nothing sexier than hearing a man moan loudly and I can only imagine the sounds of several of them all together.

[Black Caribbean British • Spiritual • <$38,000 • Bisexual/ pansexual • Single • No]

Sometimes I imagine that I am in a room with glass walls, like during interrogations where it looks like a mirror, but on the other side there is actually an audience. And men look at me and masturbate while I'm being fucked by a robot. They sometimes have control gadgets and sometimes something similar to sound-engineering equipment with which they can control the speed and actions of this robot. They often exceed the speed limit during moments of high excitement.

[Ukrainian • Atheist • <$19,000 • Bisexual/pansexual • In a relationship • No]

In my deepest sexual fantasy, I see myself in a room, naked, with the past partner I fantasise about most – it is always him. The room is darkly lit, a dreamy quality about it. I am on display. I wear nothing but a collar around my neck. He sits and I curl myself over his knees, hugging them tightly as he traces his fingers up and down my body. Without warning, he begins to spank me with his bare hand. I writhe beneath him, moaning, whimpering, getting wetter with each loud slap of his hand against my buttocks. He coos at me, praises me, tells me what a good girl I am for taking it so well. I can feel welts and bruises blossoming on my skin, and yet he continues. He works his free hand beneath my chin and slides two fingers deep into my mouth, and I feel myself slip away into a headspace I cannot define except to say I am free and floating, weightless. When he is done raining blows on my bare backside, he rubs my skin tenderly, gently massaging over the marks. He slides his fingers from my mouth and asks me what I want. My response is always the same: him, I want him. I want to be touched by him, devoured by him, used by him. I want to be his.

He guides me up from his lap with a single long digit slipped through the D-ring on my collar, pulling me up to my feet, to face him, our bodies almost in contact. He gazes down at me, letting fingers trail over my skin: against my neck, collarbones, breasts, soft tummy, round hips. He takes me in, and I can see a hunger there that makes me weak at the knees. He kisses me full on the mouth, tongue pressing just at the line of my lips, begging to be let inside. I melt into him, into his kiss, into his hard hands in my hair and at the base of my neck. We're moving, my feet shuffling backwards as he propels me with his body, and I feel something hard at my back. He breaks the kiss and grips my cheek with his fingers, turning my head to the side to look at a glass wall behind me.

As the lights come up, I realise there are dozens of faceless watchers on the other side of the glass. An audience, enraptured, watching me, watching him, watching us. I can hear quiet but excited murmurs through the glass. I steal a glance at my partner and the smirk on his mouth is unmistakable. He doesn't say a word but presses me into the glass and eases down to his knees. My heart pounds, skips a beat. He wraps his arms around me, one at the back of my thigh, hand cupping my bottom, fingers digging into the still-fresh welts he left there, the other arm dragging my other leg up over his shoulder, spreading me, allowing him to press his face full against me. He eats me like a man starved, licking, sucking, lapping at me, guzzling me down. He drives his fingers into me simultaneously, circling, come-hithering, stretching, making me ache. I arch my back and throw my neck back, allowing me to just see the heads of my audience. The energy behind me is buzzing now, a rush of murmurs, growing into a roar. I moan with abandon, fingers reaching down to wind their way through my partner's golden locks. I'm shuddering in his arms, on the verge of climax, the brightness starting behind my eyes as my knees and thighs shake. He presses his fingers inside of me like he is reaching for my orgasm, and works his tongue perfectly at the same time, and I come on his hand and mouth, my hands gripping his head fiercely as he continues to ride me with his mouth and fingers through the crest of pleasure. In my ears, blood rushing, but also the sound of thunderous applause from behind the glass.

He stands and kisses me on the mouth, letting me taste myself on his lips, before spinning me round and pressing my naked body against the glass wall, his body pressed against the back of mine. I can feel how hard he is, and I want him desperately. My mouth is open against the cold glass, almost drooling from the need I feel between my legs. The wall becomes warmer against my skin, and I realise the audience has moved closer, pressing exploratory fingers against me, against the glass. Even as they play at touching me, he is grazing his hands down my hips and thighs in real time. I feel overtaken by the sensations, my face is flushing, blushing maybe, to have so many strangers so close to my naked body while my lover is teasing me, waiting for me to beg for what I want. I give in, and a chorus of my need escapes my lips, begging him to have me right here in front of this audience. He whispers praise against my earlobe and then his hands wrap like iron around my thighs, and he pulls my legs back to smack into his, bending me at the waist, my face and arms and breasts more firmly pressed against the fragile barricade between me and my voyeurs. He teases my opening for just a second too long, reducing me once again to begging, before he forces his hips into mine and pushes his whole length inside of me. I am crying out his name as he fucks me with the expertise of a man who has known my body a thousand times, and will know it a thousand more. The familiar rhythm he knows I need. The tease, his hands feeling me, covering me, electrifying me, as I shudder and rock and whimper and moan beneath him. My audience is whispering words that are a blur to me; I cannot understand them beyond the thunder of blood in my ears. My lover's hand slides around the front of my body and his fingers move against me in time with his hips. I can feel eyes and hands all over my body, watching, whispering, I can almost feel the breath of their words. My lover is whispering my name and words of praise and encouragement and need. I can feel a fire building in my stomach, and lines of light burning around the edges of my skin. I am barely breathing, mouthing my pleasure, a chorus of the sound of my lover's name is on my lips. We come together, each exploding out of our skin at once, melting into each other, shaking, shuddering, shattered. Again, a thunderous applause, words of awe and wonder, the fleeting feeling of their touch fading away from the glass, the lights dimming, leaving us alone again. The glass transitions, inky and black for a moment, and then it becomes reflective. I see my face, slack with pleasure, skin flushed. His face comes into view as he wraps his arms around my chest, and pulls me back against him, our warm bodies burning against one another. The look of satisfaction in his eyes undoes me. He turns my face back toward his and kisses me once again, and the fantasy ends.

[White American • Atheist • >$128,000 • Bisexual/pansexual • In a relationship • No]

i always have a thing for...

Like me, you have probably been asked the age-old question: 'What is your type?' As reductive as that question always sounds, the letters in this section show that many of you most definitely like to fantasise about a very specific type of person and/or scenario.

For some, the fantasy is evidently rooted in the past, or the memory of someone they once loved or desired. For others, the notion of a particular 'thing' at the core of their arousal is much more indistinct or even amalgamated, perhaps inspired by a stranger, or a fictional character. One woman describes how uniforms for her are a classic turn-on: 'I have had sexual fantasies from as young as eight years old,' she writes. 'My first was about the postman, whom I'd imagine posting a letter to my bedroom with a big old-fashioned movie kiss for me. Since then, uniforms have always been my gateway to arousal.' For most of us, unpicking where this 'type' came from can be an emotional minefield — it might feel transgressive to fantasise about someone from the past, someone you can't have or someone you otherwise dislike, say, and maybe that's what makes it arousing.

Most of us come to accept that relationships demand compromise, but our fantasies have no such limitations. Many of the characters in these fantasies do differ wildly from the authors' real-life romantic partners. Yet there's no reason they should be seen as a threat — what we want in our fantasies isn't necessarily what we want in our real lives. A go-to fantasy can also be a one-off. One writer here even goes so far as to invite her partner into her fantasies, and they begin together to co-create their 'imaginary third', bringing storytelling into their bedroom.

I wouldn't have imagined that Agent Dana Scully in The X-Files, whom I played for much of the nineties, would have fallen into a 'type' that was considered erotic – Scully wore dowdy trouser suits and was a verified Brainiac. But of course there is the centuries-old sexy librarian trope who is imagined, once her hair is released and glasses removed, to be wild and confident under the sheets, and Scully seemed to fit neatly into this type, eliciting decades of erotic obsession and more than her share of fan fiction. More recently, when I played Prime Minister Margaret Thatcher in The Crown I was reminded by researchers that she too was something of a specific erotic type, and that there was a whole cohort of people who had a 'thing' for her – and her ankles! – despite her respectable ferocity. No doubt she was the object of a fair few of the 1980s Conservative Cabinet members' bedtime fantasies!

There is something wonderful about the perfect tailoring of the fantasies in this section and the pleasure here is most certainly in their detail. Smells, tastes, flavours and sensations; descriptions which can be intensely personal and, in some cases, obscure. Whatever someone's proclivity – be it a uniform, an encounter with a Mrs Robinson-type character, or a perfectly programmed sex robot – the hyper-specific nature of these fantasies is an integral part of their appeal.

We don't tend to question preferences for 'type' in our day-to-day, where modern life gives a bewildering amount of choice. Could it be that these fantasies are, in some way, a response to this excess of options? That what we really want is to cut to the chase with a fantasy that reliably gets us off? This could be the sexual *version of going to your favourite restaurant and ordering the same dish every time because it consistently hits the spot and always leaves you satisfied.*

•

I've always had a thing for men in a position of power, but more specifically middle-aged teachers. And for what seems like forever I've fantasised about sitting in a classroom where the teacher asks me to stay after class to discuss an overdue paper. He takes me into his office where we both pretend I don't hear him lock the door. We sit down at his desk and he looks at me briefly while reading from my paper. After a few sentences, I reach for his hand and he looks up and into my eyes with such fire and passion I feel my knees quivering. He grabs me around the neck and pulls me into a deep kiss as he lifts me up on the desk. His hands are in my hair and I desperately try to take his shirt off. He basically rips my clothes off as papers from the desk are flying around us. As he reaches my panties, he raises his mouth to mine for a long kiss before he goes down on me with such enthusiasm I've never ever been more satisfied. When he's done he picks me up and we have passionate sex up against his bookshelf. And when we're finally done, he strokes my hair and gives me one last long kiss.

[White Danish • Atheist • <$38,000 • Heterosexual • In a relationship • No]

This is a fantasy that I have had and added to over a number of years as I have matured sexually. It involves a woman slightly older than myself (forties/fifties); she is heterosexual and married or in a relationship with a man but has had curiosities about being with a woman. She is confident and has a successful career. (I've always been attracted to powerful women who have their shit together in life. For me, there is nothing more beautiful.) The woman and I meet anonymously in a hotel room with the intention of sex only. It's worth stating at the beginning that my main objective in this fantasy is for her to experience sex with a woman and to give her the most pleasure I can. I start by kissing her lips, softly first and then harder, pushing my tongue into her mouth while my hands are on her waist and moving up to her hair. I gently kiss her neck while my hands are in her hair and running down her back. I sit her on the bed and slowly start to undress her, looking into her eyes while I marvel at her beauty. Once she's naked, I take the time to kiss and stroke her body starting at the nape of her neck, down to her chest, breasts and nipples. Licking them slowly then gently biting them while my hands are digging into her hips. I move down her body, softly kissing her stomach and outer thighs, my hands grazing the backs of her legs with enough pressure from my nails for her to enjoy the sensation but not feel pain. She is now breathing heavily from anticipation but I want to make her wait before I touch her any more. I return to her mouth and kiss her deeply before I ask her where she wants me to touch her. She tells me she wants me to give her oral sex and shows me where she likes it. I kiss her inner thighs and gently suck the lips of her vulva; I part her lips and start to lick her clit slowly in long strokes. She arches her back and moans in pleasure. My strokes get faster and at the same time I slide my fingers inside deep inside her. Her breathing quickens before she orgasms while my tongue is against her clit. I feel her get wetter all over my mouth. I let her pause and I spend a while stroking her naked, warm body, not touching her sexually but letting her relax while she enjoys my touch. We're lying side by side and I kiss her hard and gently tug her hair while my hand goes up her thigh and my fingers slide inside her again. She asks me to fuck her hard with my fingers, which I do while my other hand is holding her hair. She is getting close to orgasm and I tell her to look at me while she comes. I feel her about to come while I push my fingers in deep as she climaxes and tenses around them. I take my hands off her and let her relax on the bed. I shower, kiss her softly and leave. The final part of my fantasy involves me being at a restaurant with friends, when the same woman comes in with her husband and sits on a nearby table. We share an intense moment where we alone know what we did together...

[White British • Christian • <$128,000 • Gay/lesbian • Married/ in a civil partnership • No]

During sex I have a particular fantasy I often come back to which seems to heighten and accelerate my path to orgasm. I am in period costume, a housemaid or perhaps a governess. Not highly ranked and in the employ of a household. An adult son of my employer's family returns from some kind of military expedition. We meet in the road on his way home. I wait in the back of a carriage and he enters, closing the door behind him although it doesn't lock. I pull up my skirts and he unbuttons his breeches; he's already hard and we fuck fast and breathlessly, saying how much we have missed each other. I don't know exactly what does it for me about this fantasy scenario: I think it's the outward repression of the era, the layers of period costume, the urgency, risk, the semi-public nature and feeling so desired by this hot gentleman, seeing the real, raw him and feeling him inside me, being what we each want. Anyway, it's hot as anything and works every time!

[White British • Christian • <$38,000 • Heterosexual • Married/ in a civil partnership • Yes]

I'm eighteen years old (going on nineteen), and to this day I've hardly been kissed, never mind sex and all that. It's not that I don't want it. On the contrary, I think about sex too often you might say. It takes up a lot of space in my brain. I've been masturbating since the age of nine or ten – before I even knew what the word masturbation meant, and long before I knew what an orgasm was. I just knew that it felt good.

It wasn't until I was almost twelve that I recognised that I desired women. I was sitting in the passenger seat of the car beside my mother, we were on our way to town to run errands. She had the radio on and the Rolling Stones song 'Wild Horses' was playing (I know it sounds weird) and I thought about myself, older, in bed kissing another woman. I lay in bed each night and couldn't fall asleep without thinking of being touched and caressed, kissed, open-mouthed, stripped of all my clothes by a woman.

These days I fantasise about being dominated by this woman I conceived in my head. She's a soft butch, sun-kissed skin, curly dark hair cut short. I think of her taking me in an old projection booth. I've always wanted to be fucked in a projection booth. I've snuck in with her while she's showing the film (yes, I know being a projectionist isn't a profession any more). I want her to dominate me. I want her to know all of me, for me to just surrender to her completely. She knows I'm all hers. A sex scene from an old film is showing. (*Je Tu Il Elle? Desert Hearts?*) I'm wearing my favourite yellow dress. I'm standing, watching through the square. The scene comes. And she comes up behind me. Sweeps my hair out of the way, kisses my neck, reaches for my panties. She calls me hers. I moan and whimper a little, curve my neck so I can kiss her mouth. Her tongue is against my cheek. She feels me. I'm so wet for her that I've soaked through my dress. She turns me round so we're facing each other. I'm up against the wall. She gets down on her knees and moves closer.

'*Vem amor*, I want to taste your little *maracujá*.' She spreads my legs apart, lifts up the skirt of my dress and she doesn't go right for my sex or pull off my panties. First, she teases me a little. She kisses the interior of my thighs, bites them. She runs her hands along the little stretch marks on my thighs and ass. I tell her I feel a little self-conscious about them but she tells me she loves every inch of me. She takes off my panties and runs her hand along the thick dark patch of hair. She finds my clit and sucks on it very gently. I lean my head back. It's too good. She almost bites it. And then she slips her tongue inside my cunt, and braces her hands on my ass. Her tongue is inside me. She finds my most sensitive spots. I come in her mouth. Eventually, she comes back up to me, kisses me again. 'You see how good you taste? You see why I can't resist you?' She slips her fingers inside me. I wrap my legs around her. She finds where it feels the best. And for the first time, I come from inside of myself. (I've never orgasmed from penetrative sex. I've always wanted to.) She locks eyes with me. Holds me tight. And she doesn't let go. That's the most important thing. She tells me she won't ever let go. I catch my breath for a minute. She kisses my breasts, my nipples. She says how soft I feel under her skin. She's rubbing herself against my thigh and before I know it I have her against the wall. I'm on my knees just like she was. I undo her belt and put my mouth on her sex. I love the taste of her. (I have no idea what women taste like but I can only imagine how wonderful it must be.) God. She knows I'm not as experienced as she is – so she guides me a little while praising me when I find the right places. I feel her with my hands. She's warm inside, dripping wet like me.

Another thing I think about is her wearing a strap-on. I slip my legs over her and ride her while she holds on to my hips, kisses my breasts. I want her to break me open. I want to be aware that there's little universes inside me unexplored. I don't care if it's not her sex. It's still her. Sometimes I think of being spanked and then she takes me with her strap-on, slipping it inside me until I cry out from pleasure.

The thing about this woman is that, as far as I know, she isn't real. She's only with me in my head at night, holding me while I fall asleep. And there for me in the morning. She's everything I could ever want, everything I could ever need in a person. I want this. I want her kissing my shoulders in the morning. I want her to take me dancing every Friday night. I want to make her *café con leche* in the morning. I want her to make me laugh so hard my sides hurt. I want her to hold me when I cry. I fantasise about a lot of things. Half my life has been lived inside my head. But that invisible 'she' is who I fantasise about the most. I only wish I knew her name.

[Mixed-race Brazilian American • Agnostic? • Gay/lesbian • Single • No]

It's just three lines, which I repeat to myself when I lie on my back and pull my panties to the side. My head is turned to the left and my eyes are closed as I bite my bottom lip (I read somewhere it increases the feeling in your pussy, is that true?). I frown as I try to concentrate, bring my attention back to the pulsing between my legs. (That's what they say to do in meditation, come back to the present. I'm sure more people would meditate with success if an orgasm was at the end of the tunnel.) It's been twelve years since my ex-boyfriend actually said those words, those three lines that gave me the highest orgasm of my life. But I continue to repeat them while running firm circles around my clitoris. I bite harder on my lip as I say them in my head, rocking now on my heels so that my ass rubs against the sheets.

'You like that, do you?' (Imagining his thick cock rubbing up and down on my thick lips.)

'My big hard cock making you come ...' (It enters me, stretching me open, his breath as he elongates 'c-o-o-o-m-e', warming my ear, my neck.)

'Making you moan.' (Thrusting hard, he pulls my hair to the side and bites my lip himself.)

And I do. Come. Three lines. Twelve years. One memory. Still the only way I can meditate.

[White Australian • Atheist • >$64,000 • Bisexual/pansexual • In a relationship • No]

I am an eighteen-year-old girl from the Philippines. I understand that my opinions about sex can be easily disregarded because of my age, but here I am anyway. From the age of twelve, I realised that I found both men and women attractive, though I do prefer men most of the time. I am a virgin. Growing up in a predominantly Catholic community has greatly affected the way I view femininity and sexuality, and ever since I learned how to touch myself, there's this lingering feeling of shame every time. I crave connection. Devotion, even. Sex can be such a soul-bonding experience and yet I am constantly disappointed by how disposable most women feel when it's all said and done. I'm scared now. I have a sexual preference for older men. It's a long-running joke with my friends and family but it's true and it eats me up whenever I find anybody my age even remotely attractive. It seems almost like I was meant to be this way: trying to find somebody to fill that caregiver and lover role.

My greatest fantasy is to be swept off my feet by an older man, just so I can feel desired by somebody that society would be more likely to respect. It feels insensitive to want this, because I know it's harmful to myself and disrespectful to victims of grooming. Maybe it's the thrill of doing something controversial. Immoral, even. Family vacations where I make small talk with the tourists who stumble on their words as soon as an 'exotic' girl eyes them up and down. Eye contact on the bus with the guy dressed for his nine-to-five job and smiling at him. I know perfectly well how many men would see me if they knew this. That I'm a whore or temptress or minx or slut who would absolutely deserve getting molested or harassed. That is not what I want and it's sad to know that there's a very real chance people would prove me right. I have a big heart and it's been broken again and again and all I can do is pick up the pieces and find love in places where it should not be. The tiny, tiny amount of love that is in infatuation and stolen glances. I don't know who I am yet, and I have a long way to go, but I wish, for even just a second, I could feel that somebody else looked at me like I'm more than just a friend, classmate, etc. I want someone to *see* me. I want to open up my chest and give them my soul so that only they can see it. Sex is powerful and terrifying. I don't see myself letting go of these desires any time soon. But maybe they will change, and when that day comes, hopefully it won't be because I want love, but because I already have it.

[South East Asian Filipino • Catholic • <$19,000 • Bisexual/ pansexual • Single • No]

I crave sexual attention. I'm married to a traditional conservative man. I am in my early fifties but I look like I'm in my late thirties. I hunger after the attention of men in their twenties. I want that feeling of being young and desired. I'm unable to give that up. I don't want to grow old. I don't want to shrivel. I don't want to be with someone my age. Or older. I want to be with young virile men forever. And I know I can't.

[White • Christian • >$128,000 • Heterosexual • Married/in a civil partnership • Yes]

Ageing is a peculiar thing. On the outside I look like a middle-aged woman, probably a bit too much like my mum sometimes, with greying roots and crow's feet. Inside, however, is a completely different story. My mind, my desires, my fantasies have remained unchanged since they suffered arrested development in the 1990s when I got married, aged twenty-three. My husband is the only man I have ever had sex with, but we seem to have reached a terminal hiatus (I'm not that old – I just don't want him any more) and now I must come to terms with the fact that I probably won't experience anything intimate with anyone else. I will likely die just one tiny step from virginity, but that doesn't give an accurate picture of who I am. I was, I have to say, pretty hot in my youth and fucking horny. Like, *all the time* horny.

In my fantasies I am still that younger version of me. The men I like are almost all in their mid-twenties to thirties and I have a definite type – smooth skin, good hair, lean, long-limbed bodies. I love wide, dark eyes and full lips, good teeth and strong, long-fingered hands. There is one in particular that I know from afar. He embodies perfection to me and, whoever else may occasionally 'enter the chat', he is the one I always come back to. I am safe in the knowledge that my fantasy will never be realised and can let my imagination go wherever it will – and it has taken me to some quite magnificent places.

My recurrent dream involves a beautiful boutique hotel on Lake Como and a room with French doors that open onto a Juliet balcony, overlooking the lake. I'm not sure how we got there, but I am in the hedonistic stage of tipsy and he is holding my hair back from my face as he gives me soft and sensual kisses from my eye, down to my cheek, my mouth and my neck. Gradually his hands move down my body and he starts to take off my dress. When I raise my arms, he holds them above my head and his hands are strong as he entwines my fingers through his. It is a feeling of freedom and abandon, despite his tender grasp.

Slowly, he releases his hands and they travel back down to my bare shoulders as he continues to kiss down my throat and between my breasts. Somehow, without stopping, we manoeuvre back to the bed and he lays me softly down. I reach up and pull his T-shirt over his head, revealing a smooth, toned body. I run my hands across his tightly muscled chest and shoulders and my nails scratch down his back as he kisses me harder, his mouth kissing across my breast before taking my nipple between his beautiful, pillowed lips and teasing gently with his tongue. I groan quietly with the sensation and he carries on his journey, reaching my stomach and, finally, between my legs.

He angles his knee behind mine and pushes my legs apart as he plunges his tongue deep inside me. Slowly. Lovingly. He flicks my clit with the tip of his tongue and gently nibbles and sucks. My eyes are closed and my back arched. I can feel the waves drawing in, but I try to hold back as he pauses and then I feel his cock push inside me. He has a dancer's rhythm and is generously proportioned, so my efforts to delay my orgasm become increasingly difficult. For all his youthful sensitivity, this boy knows how to fuck. He thrusts deep, hard and slow, leaning down to kiss my mouth. My hands roam his firm back, feeling the muscles bend and flex under my fingers until we simultaneously reach the heights of ecstasy. I feel his breath stutter as he comes. We stay like that for a minute, holding the moment between us. Then he lies propped beside me, stroking my face and my hair. Through the night we talk, still naked, but sitting wrapped in a blanket in front of the open doors as the cool lake breeze wafts over us. We eventually fall asleep at dawn, my head on his chest and his arms around me.

Later we venture out to a restaurant. We find a small trattoria and bag a table in a shadowy corner, sitting beside one another. We eat bowls of pasta with fresh baby tomatoes and sip cold glasses of wine as we talk and kiss intermittently until he leans across to draw my attention to two women at a table on the other side of the restaurant, talking low, their heads close. I look closer and glance below the tablecloth – one is quietly fingering the other.

He leans in to kiss me, his white teeth gently biting my bottom lip and his hand finding its way between my legs. His fingers loop in beneath my underwear, their tips just brushing me intimately. We throw some money on the table and he pulls me out of the restaurant into the dark and quiet street, no words spoken but both of us knowing exactly what we want. We duck into a side alley where he pushes me up against the wall, kissing me hard on the mouth. I tug at his belt and open his jeans as he deftly pulls my underwear aside and we fuck, his hips pushing hard against me. I have one leg wrapped behind his thighs and my hands on his arse as he thrusts deep, kissing me deeper. It doesn't take long to climax, and I don't care if anyone can see us. He is everything I have ever wanted and I feel no shame. I am proud.

[White British • Catholic • <$64,000 • Heterosexual • Married/in a civil partnership • Yes]

Pretty much all of my fantasies have roots in my history. Most involve the pain of betrayal. This one is my favourite.

I have booked a mani pedi to come to the house, but I'm held up at work and rather than be charged for no service my boyfriend says he will take the appointment. He's never had either before and the whole thing makes him laugh. He's nervous. More so when a gorgeous twenty-something walks through the door. She puts him at ease by saying she does men's nails all the time, that he should sit back on the sofa and relax. She fills a tub with warm sudsy water and kneels on the floor to gently place his feet in it. Her thin skirt rides up her tanned legs and as she bends he can see down her blouse – she's not wearing a bra. He literally can't believe his luck. She takes one of his hands in hers and turns it over to look at his nails. After placing a towel on his lap she starts working on them with a clipper and a file. She is kneeling before him with his hand in hers – and it's legal.

He awkwardly asks how many she does a day. Where she is from. Does she enjoy it? She answers in a soft confident voice and then works in silence, one finger at a time as he watches, speechless and astonished that this beautiful woman is touching him. He stares at her hair, her smooth shoulders, her lips. She might just be the most beautiful woman who has ever paid attention to him.

When she is done filing and shaping the nails on both hands, she squirts cream into his palms and begins to massage, gently but firmly up to his elbow and back down again; in between his fingers, kneading his palms. He can see her nipples through her blouse. He is in heaven. He starts to get hard. He knows that it's showing just inches from where she is working. He is mortified. He shifts his free arm to hide it. He can't look at her. 'It's ok,' she says, 'it happens all the time.'

'It does?!' he says and apologizes.

'Don't worry,' she says, as she places his hands in his lap and moves on to his feet, taking each one out of the tub and drying them gently with the towel. As she places one of his feet on her bare thigh and starts inspecting his nails she says, 'People pay me extra.'

'I'm sorry?' he says.

'They pay me extra for extra things.'

'Like what?' he says nervously as she starts to clip and then file his toenails.

'Some pay me to do this topless, others pay me to do it entirely naked.' My boyfriend can't quite believe what he's hearing. He can't believe what has landed on his doorstep. His breathing quickens. She continues: 'And some people pay me to finish them off.' He shifts his weight on the sofa, attempting to relieve the pressure of his erection pulsing against his jeans.

'It doesn't bother you?' he says.

'Noooo!' she says. 'I like seeing what happens to people when I kneel at their feet.' She smiles mischievously and locks eyes with him. 'Do you want me to take my shirt off?' My boyfriend stutters, he has no idea what to say but before he can utter a sound, she has taken her shirt off. 'It's on me,' she says, 'you're cute.' He stares at her beautiful small breasts and plump nipples, his hand absentmindedly moving to his bulging cock. 'You can touch yourself, I don't mind,' she says. He stares deep into her eyes, did she really just say that? He allows his gaze to move over her beautiful form, her luscious hair, her soft skin, as he slowly undoes his button, unzips his jeans and places his hand over his throbbing erection. 'That's better,' she says as she squirts cream on her hands and begins to massage his feet, pressing her thumbs into his soles and rubbing her fingers in and out between his toes. He can't stand it. He's never been so turned on. She moves to his other foot, clipping and filing. He reaches under his briefs and starts stroking harder. He swears she is pressing his heel into her crotch while she files. He is so close to coming. She squirts cream on his foot and starts to dig in, again her fingers between his toes. So fucking sexy. His hand is fully on his cock now, stroking up and down, faster and faster, he's about to explode. And before he knows it, she has moved herself between his legs, pushed his hand out of the way, and is lowering her plump lips and wet mouth all the way down to the hilt. Up and down, deeper and deeper, wetter and wetter as her fingers slide over his balls. He thinks his head might explode but then suddenly she is up on her haunches, pulling her panties to the side as she slides her soaking wet pussy onto his shaft, her head inches from his, her hair falling over his face. She locks her dark brown eyes onto his and moves expertly up and down his throbbing cock, her firm thighs pressing against his sides. He wraps his mouth around one of her nipples and sucks and licks gently while she rubs her fingers against her clit and continues to grind. He looks up into her eyes as she lowers her mouth onto his and her tongue deep into his throat, faster and faster, deeper and harder and faster, until they both explode together.

An hour later, I get home. No sign of any of it. My boyfriend has showered. It was fine, he says. But for a change, he's made me dinner.

[White American • None • Pansexual • In a relationship • Yes]

I can't wait for perfectly built, fully realistic, sexually functioning male robots. I have a strong technology background and I know this will happen – long after female robots appear, but they will. Perhaps once the market for female sex robots is saturated (do pardon the pun). I also know this likely won't occur within my lifetime, or at least until well after my interest in sex has waned.

I imagine I would keep my robots in a special large, walk-in storage space, where I could unreservedly explore my sexuality with them in absolute safety and privacy. Robots are necessary for this fantasy because a group of real men could never focus on a woman sufficiently to participate, much less an individual man. (Our planet is in a primitive state. The male ego bullies the female ego – and that's that. It's a worldwide phenomenon and the prevailing state for all of recorded history. The sexual revolution has been great and I'm super glad I've seen it – but when you look at the big picture, not only is it a drop in the pan, affecting only a small number of women, but its duration within a historical context is a blip, and there are strong indications of backlash – and there's absolutely no logical reason to simply assume any gains will last. If in doubt, please refer to the conservative elements at play in current politics, which show strong signs of attempting to start a new 'Gilead'.)

SO – what would I do with my robots?! I would, of course, program them to execute my sexual fantasies. I'd create a playlist with roles and scenarios and call up the fantasy and players depending on my mood. For example, I have many fantasies involving multiple men making love to me in many different scenarios. I'm their teacher, or a babysitter who arrives to babysit – the wife isn't home and the group of men about to leave decide to stay and play with me instead.

The robots are all wonderful lovers; their greatest pleasure is to pleasure me. They will know what this means because I'll have provided instructions! I could go on and on and on about the actual fantasies ... I masturbate thinking of them all the time. I'd use them to pleasure me one-on-one as well. When I say realistic, I really mean it — I feel their throbbing penises as they come (when I want them to) and the warmth of their ejaculate inside me.

My very fondest wish is that men will read this and be utterly astonished. And possibly face their fear. Exactly what are they afraid of? And what, for that matter, are women afraid of? It's all so wasteful and ridiculous. It is so sad that the planet is in such a primitive state.

[White Canadian • Buddhist • >$64,000 • Heterosexual • Single • Yes]

I have had sexual fantasies from as young as eight years old. My first was about the postman, whom I'd imagine posting a letter to my bedroom with a big old-fashioned movie kiss for me. Since then, uniforms have always been my gateway to arousal; the male pin-ups in my mind are doctors, firefighters, sailors, soldiers, even park rangers. Perhaps I'm just so full of gratitude for these resourceful, brave and compassionate souls that I want to make love to them all. Yes, and sometimes, all at once.

During the pandemic, I started to talk very openly with my husband about who I thought of while we were making love in our bedroom. Just as I orgasm, it's often the broad-shouldered soldier with the greasy brown shoulder-length hair down between my thighs, not him, as I lie on his canvas flysheet between missile attacks, while the rest of his squad watch from their bunks. Astonishingly, my husband's face became radiant with lust at my honesty. I felt empowered and delighted when he asked me to describe more. Consequently, exploring and playing with the idea of having a 'third' in our relationship has become a fascinating, evolving sexual fantasy. The following is our most recent scenario, told as closely as it is in our bedroom. We call it Billy the Third.

Our fallen soldier arrives unexpectedly one dark, frosty morning. Our contract is to make him happier. I open the door, and he removes his threadbare khaki balaclava. He doesn't say hello, but I do and usher him in. He walks straight through, doesn't remove his rancid boots, and finds my husband. They shake hands, and I walk along the hallway inhaling the kerosene and gunmetal smell he left trailing behind him. I offer him toast from the kitchen counter (we hadn't got round to assembling the new dining table in time). He ignores the toast and asks to walk with my husband. They come home an hour later with a rainbow trout; my husband delights in telling me that Billy caught it with his bare hands. Billy prepares the fish with the penknife from his pocket, and he doesn't mind me standing there watching him cook it. He splits it three ways, and we eat in silence.

When we finish, Billy asks why branches are covering the lawn, and I tell him we haven't cleared them since the storm. He goes out and starts a fire using just garden debris and the flint and steel from around his neck. While I wash plates, my husband asks if I'm happy taking Billy in, and I tell him, rather blissfully, that I'm still taking him in. I'm so impressed by him that I wonder if there is anything he can't do, I say. My husband laughs and reminds me that he can't smile. Before we retire to bed, we notice that Billy isn't in the spare bedroom. Instead, he's on the floor, screwing the new dining-room table together. My husband is in just a pair of Bshetr underpants, and I'm commando in my black silk bed slip, but we climb over and try to help him with the job.

When it's done, Billy settles in the corner, his knees up to his chest, mud speckling the leather of his boot soles. We sit down on either side of him, then he shows us his cock, which is longer and pinker and wider and shinier than any I have ever seen before. It is a saintly stake of flesh that points to the heavens, aloof and destined to do good. He gives it a few soft strokes, and I see some pre-come glisten on his head. I jump onto the new table, open my legs, and play with my vagina. I feel two tongues take hold of my clitoris and anus, which makes me feel so slippery and wet. After minutes I'm on the edge of an orgasm, so I ask for more, and Billy hovers over me, his dog tag dangling in my face, delving his cock deep into my vagina while my husband enters my anus. The feel of their sliding girths rubbing together through my sopping dividing wall is eye-spinning. I come. I writhe around the table, clutch at my tits and feel free. Both sit back down next to each other, cocks in hand. Then I take both

of their penises into my giddy mouth to delight at their smiles
looking back at me.

*[White British • Pagan • <$38,000 • Heterosexual • Married/in a
civil partnership • Yes]*

gently, gently

'Hands and mouths moving soft and slow ...'

I n reading these letters, I've come to see that there is no one type of fantasy, just like there is no one typical 'woman'. What we want in our sex lives is as various as what we want from work, from our relationships and from love. We are all different, we all contain multitudes.

So far in this book we've witnessed a whole universe of wildly imagined adventures and scenarios which couldn't be further removed from reality. However, we also received a number of letters that spoke of just wanting to feel seen, expressing a desire for romance, affection and softness, and a longing for a strong connection to another person. 'Is it crazy that my wildest sexual fantasy is to feel safe?' reads one letter. For some, this seemingly simple desire may well be very far from their everyday reality. This yearning is reflected not only in actions but in geographical surroundings too, the fantasies often taking place in forests and gardens. Some letters mention water or bathing and an accompanying sensation of warmth, of being sensually surrounded or engulfed. There's a strong sense of wanting to return to basics, uncomplicated by the complexities and whirlwind of modern life, to ground oneself in and feel a connection with Mother Earth.

There is also a yearning in some women here for safety and comfort as a result of sexual abuse. One woman's ultimate fantasy is 'to be mothered', which makes me wonder to what extent her fantasy might serve to heal the damage of an early trauma. In other letters, a desire for tenderness clearly springs from the profound loneliness of a sexual relationship that lacks emotional intimacy. These fantasies often get to the heart of sexual appetite: emotional attachment, for these women, is a necessity for sexual arousal. One woman, for example, longs for 'Eye contact throughout, to portray the deep emotions from within. The desire, the connection, the adoring love. There must be love there, no one-night stand, no drunken lust, just love.'

Every successive generation of women has become more independent, but these letters show that, for some, this coexists with a desire to be dependent: to be cared for, soothed, stroked and affirmed. The intensity of connection described here ultimately reveals a longing for someone's undivided care and attention, both physically and emotionally. Perhaps this desire has intensified the more hyperconnected our world has become. It's pretty obvious that technology and smartphones vie for our attention to the detriment of our real-life relationships sometimes. Physical proximity is no longer a guarantee of meaningful time together. We can be in touch with people all around the world through our devices, but these same tools can be a barrier to the intimacy of in-person connection, and in fact statistics show that no matter where you live or how long you have been in a relationship, people are lonelier than ever.

One of the best pieces of advice uttered in Sex Education was not from my character, Dr Jean Milburn, but from her son Otis, played by Asa Butterfield (albeit written by creator Laurie Nunn). He said, 'It's time to stop passively hearing and start actively listening.' An old soul in a Gen Z body. I think that what we'd learn is what the letters in this section ultimately testify; that what all human beings want is to be loved, to have our basic needs met, and to be treated with kindness, gentleness and respect, not only in our sexual lives but in our day-to-day lives as well.

•

I'm almost too scared to write this, an articulation of the need that fills me with embarrassment. An inadequate fantasy. So small and insignificant, pathetic almost, yet writing it down in black and white fills me with terror; it somehow means I *own* this need, as ridiculous as that seems. So, what fantasy, what profound revelation can engender such hideously conflicting feelings? Simply this: I want to be kissed. Kissed on the lips, gently, roughly with passion, once again before I am no more.

[White British • Atheist • >$128,000 • Gay/lesbian • Single • Yes]

Whenever he enters my thoughts, I give in and my ADHD helps me zone out entirely from wherever I am and straight into his bed, over a kitchen counter, wherever. A thought of him, holding my neck tightly while I climax with his fingers deep in me – it might occur at the dentist's office, while I wait for my child to get her teeth checked.

In my mind he has a name, inspired by an emotion that cannot entirely be explained in one word. It's a box of feelings he carries to me in his veiny hands every time he and I come together. In front of him, I don't ever feel 'naked' – I feel liberated, alive. He is a good listener, better than my husband. After we confide our deepest desires to each other, we feel closer than ever before and it is almost as if I see how opening up to our vulnerabilities lets our fluids in. We lean in, we lick each other's faces, body parts, and cuddle like two cats, wet and comfortable. Our mouths stop moving but the talk between us never stops. It switches from portal to portal, begins with my voice and ends with his touch. I lose my boundaries. When he tells me to grab his cock and hold it tightly while he licks my face, I lose my pre-built status and drop the motherhood chains. Whenever I decide not to listen to what he wants, he asks me to do something else; and when he sees I don't want something, he does precisely what he knows I like. He puts his fingers deep inside me, holds my neck, speaks to me kindly through the warmth of his breath and tells me only truths. I already know that I don't have the nicest smile in the world – my teeth are small, my gums are high, but he licks both while telling me that my flaws turn him on. When he speaks these truths to me I hear it differently than from my own voice. While I climax, and I always do during this part, he holds me tighter and closer to himself and my fingers run through his short hair. Then he lies next to me, tells me how lovely that was, asks nothing of me. That turns me on, him asking nothing of me, just holding me as I rest and regain strength. Every orgasm with him drains me, I feel light and lifted. I feel like a different person, one who doesn't have her day on repeat, waking up early, preparing my kid for school and going to work. Filling the fridge, cleaning the house. Walking the dog, paying the rent. I feel released ... awakened. His smells trigger me in ways I would never be triggered. I always ask him not to wash before we meet, because his smells make me come faster. Me ... who always asked men before him to take a shower. He smells like my fingers after they've been in my own pussy, naughty and comforting. I reach for his cock and I talk to it gently, with a slight smile, and by allowing me, he lets me know that he likes it. I tell his dick how important it is to me and how for many days after we meet I feel full. His cock grows erect and I take him into my mouth, deep and slow. I go all the way, I know I can with him and that feels so safe. I spit on him and talk to him gently, I caress him and pet him, grasp it tightly and enjoy the life that fills it. Everything is slippery and I love it.

He ejaculates and I don't care: I am full, satisfied and I love him purely without any expectations. Liberated. I come near his face, meet his eyes and give him a wet, smelly kiss on a cheek.

The dentist calls me in, the check-up is finished. He praises me for my child's clean teeth and I tell him I am doing my best.

[Serbian • Atheist • <$64,000 • Heterosexual • Married/in a civil partnership • Yes]

Touch. Intimate touch. Not just a brush or brief contact but a long, drawn-out touch, skin on skin. Eye contact throughout, to portray the deep emotions from within. The desire, the connection, the adoring love. There must be love there, no one-night stand, no drunken lust, just love. It's all anyone wants. And in the confirmation of that love through sexual contact and pleasure, you find peace and brief glimpses at what it truly means to be alive. And that is human connection.

[African American and White • Mormon (dabble in paganism) • <$19,000 • Bisexual/pansexual • Single • No]

My hope: to be touched. I am fifty and no one likes to touch me. I'm tired of working to make a better self, if all the work I do is only that I accept not to be touched by anyone. It looks like I'll have to spend the rest of my life without caresses or anyone who wants to have fun with me and my excitement. If my man doesn't even like to touch me, the man who knows and loves me, how could there be anybody else? So, this is my secret dream, to be touched, to have fun in bed with somebody who likes to give me joy.

[Swiss • <$128,000 • Heterosexual • In a relationship • No]

Every time I have sex, I'm generally heavily intoxicated or under the influence of drugs. I completely freeze in fear and dissociate, even when I don't want to. Even if it's been with a friend, I still can't bring myself to mentally be there. I don't find sex to be a fun experience, it doesn't feel good, and I can't figure out why I feel so different from everyone else in the world. But there is a part of me deep down that wants more than anything to be loved, to have filthy, hot and sensual sex. Whether it be from a man, woman, non-binary, etc.

My sexual fantasy would be something beautiful, loving and safe. I want to fall into bed with someone I TRUST, who won't hurt me, who won't use me. I fantasise about actually having FUN while having sex, it feeling GOOD. Of someone who appreciates my body and truly loves it. I don't want to be thinking about how fat I am or how I'm not good enough, or experienced enough. I just want to be truly loved. I want to feel good enough. I'd say if I dug even further in my mind, my ultimate sexual fantasy would be a combination of the above with a bit of kink. A bit of choking, a bit of dirty talk and a bit of roughness. Because who doesn't want a little bit of a thrill? But again, I want those things with guaranteed safety and love. I'd love someone to throw me onto the bed and make my legs quake, like I read in the smut novels. To be bent over the kitchen counter and taken right then and there because someone loves me so much they need me in that moment. Is it crazy that my wildest sexual fantasy is to feel safe?

[White American • Spiritual • <$38,000 • Bisexual/pansexual • Single • No]

I am in a small valley in the countryside, far away from humans. I slowly undress, take deep breaths, and let the air play with my nipples and clitoris. I carefully select little twigs and leaves and touch my clit with them softly as I lie on the ground with my legs spread apart, letting the sun and the air travel across my body and warm my insides, as well as my outside. Then I start rubbing myself against the moist soil, smelling the freshness and purity of it. I pause and take deep breaths as I lie there, fully covered in mud. The lust is becoming unbearable. I quickly put my underwear back on and head to a nearby tree. I start kissing, licking and pressing my vagina against its uneven surface, desperately trying to warm up the tree's core and make it feel what I feel, make it share what I share. I moan loudly, a shout-out to Mother Nature, grateful for everything that she gave me, grateful for my mind and body, which now is solely devoted to her.

[Greek • Atheist • <$19,000 • Bisexual/pansexual • Cohabiting • No]

A recent fantasy, forged from dream fragments: I'm in the woods. I am lost, but not scared, only curious. There is a path, and I know I will find my way. As I walk, I become aware that I am being watched. The trees seem to have eyes, even as the forest seems to have hushed. My senses are heightened. I hear every brush of branch across its neighbour; the subtle breeze brings goose bumps to my arms. The lush and lively forest smell rises to my nostrils. The moss looks inviting, the ferns' curls beckon. Everything feels alive. A figure appears before me; he almost seems to materialise from the air. My watcher. I recognise him as Bigfoot; not a monstrous apeman, but a tall, powerful figure covered in soft fur with a strong jaw. He exudes confidence, with a gentleness. He knows who he is and what he can be. He's observing me, taking me in, as I do him. I know he is here for me. I am drawn to him. He has green eyes with flecks of brown; eyes that reflect the forest itself. He moves toward me. He walks on two legs, but has the crouching fluidity of a deer or mountain lion. I see the soft sex organs hanging between his legs, the way his fur fades around them. His penis is naked but protected. He is larger than any man I've known, and looks like an animal, but he's completely non-threatening. He is curious and open, like I am. Once our eyes lock, I feel woozy, cocooned in this soft green space. Everything has changed. My path is to him. In one fluid motion he places a massive hand behind my head, leans in and kisses me. His mouth engulfs mine. We are locked together by our lips, and I feel the lick of desire thickening and extending through me. My body bends into his without resistance or effort. I am easily swept into his arms as he holds me, legs around his waist, my body pressed against him. He holds me effortlessly in one arm as he peels off my clothes with the other. The feeling of his soft fur and crisp forest air against my bare skin emboldens me, and I reach my arms around him, no longer passive but insistent, needy. My fingers tangle in his fur and I rub my breasts against him, feeling his softness. I grind my pelvis against him, the heat rising throughout my body. I am weightless in his arms and writhe, aware that I am performing, which takes me out of my body enough for me to realise that my performance is being appreciated by the eyes of others in the woods. I see myself from the outside, I see my naked need on display, I feel it from within, and then I feel my Bigfoot's cock against me as he lowers my body down his: it is large and hard, rising from his fur; my ass and pussy ride on top of it, slick and teasing me between my legs. A few more movements, and his large cock enters me, completely filling me, and while it doesn't hurt, every small motion sends a ripple through me as if every nerve has been dipped in fire. But it's not just his cock: his genitals extend beyond his penis and I feel part of him grow and extend into a new member, something smaller than his cock: it presses against my ass, entering me and pulsing softly. And on my clitoris — not a mouth, exactly, but a beautiful swelling that surrounds and attaches to my clitoris, and with these three instruments he plays every string of desire, every chord of pleasure in my body. We are fused together and our motions move and swirl like water, and it's more than fucking, it's an integration. I am an animal, his animal, but also rising within myself to be a howl, a divining rod of pleasure in nature, an energetic masterpiece. I realise he has been holding me all this time as I have felt weightless. I look into his eyes and push on his shoulders; he reads my signal. He bends his legs and lies back on the ground so I am straddling him. I want his weight on top of me, I want to feel this magnificent beast hold me down and take me, but I know he wants me to be seen. And I want this too, to be exactly where I am, straddling his strong body, my legs wide over his hips as his magical pelvis works its fire in me, around me. While I ride him, I learn that even as I lift my hips and swirl and dance my cunt on him, his animal organs move with me in a rhythm that builds a deep pleasure that feels multidimensional. It is all-encompassing. I move and draw his power into me and my energy is boiling and shoots into the forest around me. I imagine he's reached all the way through me to massage my heart. The shock of this new feeling keeps me from coming even though the pleasure is making me gasp and groan. My curiosity once again extends to the woods around me. The eyes in the woods – are they Bigfoots? Wolves? Or wolfmen? Wolf-people? They are watchful and lusty; they growl softly in a chorus of desire that echoes in my ears. They all want to see me come.

I look into my Bigfoot's eyes as my attention collapses back into our bodies, his tension between my thighs as I squeeze his cock in me. I feel his soft furry hands on my breasts and back. I pinch his large nipples and bend to suckle one, my body an arc of desire, of taking and giving. He cups my ass strongly in both hands and urgently quickens his motions, his hips thrusting up into me. It's so much, I'm full, I'm bursting, and I lose sense of the edges of my body as pleasure courses through me. Just when I think my orgasm will subside, it builds again, and I'm shaking, so much that my eyes tear up and the aftershocks roil through to my very edges: my fingertips, my hair follicles, a trickle down my spine. Only when my throat quiets do I realise I've been moaning. Howling? My Bigfoot smiles at me, he too is out of breath. His penis and extended sexual organs soften and release me. I lie back in the moss: warm, sticky, humming with joy. A rustle in the brush and ferns around me and those who have been patiently watching emerge from the forest. The soft yet piercing eyes grace the noble faces of strong lithe bodies. The wolf-people approach on all fours, exuding protection and safety and desire. They surround me, lie against me, and use gentle paws to roll me over and play with my limbs. They use their noses to nuzzle me and their long tongues to lick me clean before nudging me into a foetal position. My Bigfoot, meanwhile, has gathered foliage and built a nest. I fall asleep in a puppy pile of fur, my face pressed into the warm and gently rising chest of my Bigfoot, his wolves curled around us, warm, safe, exhausted.

[White American • Atheist • <$19,000 • Bisexual/pansexual • Married/in a civil partnership • Yes]

My deepest sexual fantasies can be summed up by what I like to call 'Care Play'. I have general fantasies and one specific one that I play out in my mind when I can't sleep at night and if porn or my Wank Bank (my secret 'spicy' album of pictures and gifs) just aren't doing it. I should preface this by stating that I've only had one actual 'long' relationship and I've never actually gotten to do any of these things. Mostly because I never felt that my partner would be willing and also because I felt like they were a lot to ask.

This fantasy is super-nerdy so just be ready for that. It sounds silly and I feel a bit of shame while I'm typing this out, but here goes:

I'm at a magical university in Scotland, so basically Hogwarts, but I'm an adult, like I am now because the whole 'underage student with a teacher' thing is super-creepy and problematic. Anyways, it's like a big castle where the students are all residents, like a boarding school, and the professors live in too. The fantasy always starts with me just wandering the castle because I can't sleep. I walk by a few of my favourite classrooms, hoping the smells of potions, old books and wood will lull me to sleep. I walk by my favourite professor's room and hear his footsteps. His footsteps stop and I can tell he's heard me wandering around. His door opens softly and he looks at me in a way that says he's not surprised to see me at this time of the night. He asks if I can't sleep and says he can't either and, if I have a few minutes, that he can make a potion.

He pulls down a cauldron and taps it with his wand and blue flames emerge from under it. I can hear the sound of liquid filling up and he asks me to get the blue tin with gold stars from the shelf above his desk and I do as I'm asked. I bring it back to him and set it near his hands. I look at them and they're rough, worn, scarred, but still somehow strong. I like them. I like how much bigger his hands are than mine. He catches me looking at them and seems a bit amused. Next, he asks me to fetch two mugs from under the cupboard near his leg while he starts pouring whatever was in the tin into the cauldron. I realise he could be doing all this by magic and that he just wants me to feel useful.

He asks why I can't sleep and if this is normal for me. I'm about five years older than most of the other students in my year and he knows this but I'm not sure if he knows why I have had a late start at this university. I tell him I was in the military and went through some things that keep me up at night. I have night terrors and don't like to wake the others in my corridor, so I usually wander around until I'm too tired to have any fight left in me to make noises in my sleep. He looks at me like he understands, instead of the usually confused or pitiful look I'm familiar with. He hands me some chocolate from his sweater pocket and a bit sternly says, 'Eat. You'll feel better.'

Something stirs inside me. He tells me that he's seen things that keep him awake too, that he's done things he's not proud of but that he wouldn't change the past even if he could because it put him where he is now. As he talks the potion starts to fill the room with an amazing aroma of fresh clean sheets, pine, cigar smoke and the smell of sunshine on your skin. I ask him what it is and he tells me it's what he calls his 'Sleepy Time Tea': a potion that makes you feel calm and safe. He asks me what I smell and I tell him. There's another smell that I just can't place until he steps closer. It's him. It's the smell of his sweater, chocolate and the metallic smell of cauldrons that fill his classroom. I suddenly feel as if he heard that last thought and turn away.

When he hands me the mug of potion his hands linger on mine. I take a sip of the tea and it's perfect. I suddenly feel calmer than I've felt in years and put my head on his chest while hugging him. He tenses up at my touch and I freeze, but then his shoulders relax and I hear him set his cup down and he wraps his arms around me. I tell him thank you in a small voice but he understands how much it means to me. He runs his hand over the back of my head and I look up at him. I stand on my tiptoes to reach his lips and wait for him to meet me the rest of the way. He hesitates but then meets my lips. His hand slips down to my neck and he uses it to push our faces apart a bit and just looks down at me. This time I see joy. I nod and he knows I'm OK with moving forward.

He lifts me up and places me on his desk. Moving his hands further down. He slows down when he reaches my chest and lifts my shirt off, kissing my chest and neck softly but a bit fast. He stops again and just takes the sight of me sitting on his desk all in. He asks if this is what I want and when I say 'Yes, sir,' he gets a sort of wild excited grin on his face. He grabs his wand and points it towards what I believed was a small cupboard and the door opens up. He carries me through, still kissing my neck and chest. The walls are lined with books, specimens in jars and candles, and again he flicks his wand and the room begins to fill with warmth and candlelight. I look up and a crescent moon is shining down on us. There's a small bed, and he sets me down on it and begins to take his layers off. I quickly help him and he helps me to remove the rest of my clothes. He looks at me and touches me softly and I yawn. The Sleepy Time Tea is kicking in and I don't want it to. He says it's OK if I'm sleepy and that we can just take it slow for today. I tell him I'm sorry but he just tells me that he understands and that he'd be in the same boat if he'd had time to actually drink the tea as well, laughing at how fast I made my move. I drift off with my head on his chest listening to his heartbeat. I start to watch the scene as if I'm a picture on the wall and I see him running his hand through my hair, holding me tighter when I wriggle in my sleep, telling me I'm OK and I'm safe with him. Slowly, he falls asleep too and the fantasy ends.

Most of my fantasies are just me wanting to feel safe and taken care of. I'm very into sex but I'm more into the before and after. I love when men take time to make me feel like they care about building trust. This is my deepest desire.

[Mixed Hispanic/Native American • Spiritual • <$64,000 • Heterosexual • Single • No]

It feels like I'm admitting to some kind of failure by saying this, but: I want to be mothered. I fear this makes me the worst cliché of what they say about lesbians; that some signals got crossed in my addled lesbian brain and now I want a slightly older woman to take care of me and hold me and then, yes, also have sex with me gently, patiently, until I can learn to trust her and relax and let it be an adventure again.

I want this woman's fingers tangled in my hair and tracing my breasts, and while she does that, I want a cocoon to form around us and shield us so that no bad news can reach us. I want to feel safe from the outside world, from pending catastrophes. I want my mind to quiet (it never quiets, even in my best memories of sleepy sex). In bed, I always find that part of me is somewhere else – maybe it's back in the homophobia of my upbringing, or the purity culture of the church, or stuck reliving the last crisis while simultaneously preparing for the next one. I want to feel wholly myself when we are having sex and I want to really, fully *be* there. What I want feels hard to even put into words. What is it like to be present during sex and enjoy all the parts of it and not have to engage in the 'but what does she really want' dance, swimming in our two lifetimes of shame that merge every time we touch? What's it like for sex to be an exploratory game, fun that isn't rushed, pleasure that we have a lifetime to discover? What if our sex was a home that welcomed us back, again and again, yet different every time? Celebrated as its own peaceful joy instead of it working overtime as a Band-Aid to solve something else?

She is older and surer of herself than me. Her quiet confidence will guide me to reach into myself to find my real desires instead of another young queer woman's panicky doubts compounding with mine. I want to explore with her. I think this fantasy scenario I'm describing is simply one without fear. Because fear is baked into me in so many ways – fear of having sex, fear of having sex with a woman, fear of what I want, fear of enjoying it, or of hating it. Of my body. Perhaps of my actual mother, yes. Fear of hurting my partner and fear of them hurting me. I see this fear wrapped around me like a wispy, solid spider's web, and as I lie there in bed with this older woman, it gets softly lifted up and it floats away. Here, I can trust my body and its wishes. The woman trusts hers, too.

[White American • Atheist • <$64,000 • Gay/lesbian • Single • No]

I was sexually assaulted when I was eleven and it deeply affected my view of sex and sexuality for a very long time. When adolescence came, I had 'boyfriends' and crushes, and desperately wanted to explore intimacy and sex with them, but when faced with an actual opportunity, I would shut down in terror and panic. At a time when my friends were 'rounding the bases', I avoided all sexual or intimate contact. I didn't have my first kiss until I was nineteen, was twenty-one or twenty-two when I first had oral sex, and didn't lose my virginity until I was twenty-seven. I went through with almost all of my sexual encounters because I felt like I was a freak and I didn't want to be 'broken' any more – none of the men were particularly attentive and not only did I not have an orgasm, but in some cases I totally dissociated during the whole experience. At the same time, my sex drive was always very high and I would masturbate regularly, often daily. I read erotica and had a very rich fantasy life.

My fantasies have almost always centred around a very caring, supportive man – he's usually faceless. I am very attracted to him for many reasons but most important is that I trust him. He touches me slowly, gently, and talks to me; about how he loves me and my body; how much he wants me; how much he wants to make me come with his hands, his mouth and his cock. He wraps me in his arms and kisses me so deeply, hands caressing but always checking to see if I'm comfortable or how I'm feeling. He looks at me with such reverence and lust, as if I were his fantasy come to life. He undresses me and touches each new sliver of skin; he asks me to take his hands in mine and show him where and how I like to be touched. He keeps talking to me, telling me how good I feel, how sexy I am, what he wants me to feel, and how he feels. His words stay soft but become dirtier and more urgent as he becomes more and more aroused. He takes my hands to show me how he wants me to caress his body and stroke his cock, and he praises me when I touch him in a way that he likes. He fingers me while looking at my face and then whispers about how wet I am and how much he wants to taste me. He kisses down my body to my pussy and starts to eat me out, all the while looking at my face and checking in to see that I'm OK with everything that is happening. I come hard on his fingers and mouth and he kisses back up my body, letting me taste myself on his lips. I tell him how much I want and need him inside me, how much I want to feel his cock in me, his come in me. He looks deeply into my eyes as he pushes inside of me, taking his time and rubbing my clit as I am so tight, helping my body to relax and take him in. Again, he talks to me – about how wet and tight I am, how good I feel around him. How much he wants me to come around his cock. His fingers are stroking my clit and he's kissing my breasts and neck, whispering to me how good I am, how much he loves being inside me and fucking me. How much he wants me to come, to see my face when I let go. He tells me I'm beautiful and sexy, and strong. He feels me start to go over the edge and rubs a gentle but insistent pattern on my clit, watching me as I come. He tells me that he loves watching me come, loves feeling my pussy tighten around his cock, how much he wants to fill me with his come. I tell him I want to feel him come inside me and he begins to chase his own orgasm, fucking into me harder but still looking at me, still connecting and telling me how good it feels to fuck me. I feel him start to come inside me and I touch myself and come again while he is still inside me. He rolls over so I can lie on his chest, and we kiss and laugh. His cock slips out of me and I feel his come dripping out. He tells me he can't wait until he can be inside of me again; how he wants us to talk about our biggest fantasies and try things we're curious about. I tell him I want to suck his cock and have him come all over my tits. He tells me he wants to watch me with my vibrator and learn how I make myself come. He draws us a warm bath and we sit, wrapped up in each other, kissing lazily.

He dries me off and takes me to the bed where we fall asleep in each other's arms. I know that he will be there when I wake up and I fall asleep listening to his heartbeat.

[White American • Agnostic • <$128,000 • Heterosexual • Single • Yes]

I have always been sex-positive. Recently, though, I've come to realise that I do not feel sexual attraction the way other people do. Actually, I don't feel sexual attraction at all. I do, however, thoroughly enjoy having sex. You can see how this would cause conflict in myself ... So, I'll tell you what an asexual like me dreams about when my partner is out of town or too tired.

It always starts with me lying on my bed, my body exposed and vulnerable. I close my eyes, allowing the thoughts to take over, and soon I get lost in a world of my own imagination. In my fantasy, I am the object of desire, and all eyes are on me. I'm wearing a tight red dress that accentuates my curves in all the right places, and I feel so beautiful. I can feel the heat of the eyes as I walk through the room, as if I'm an animal in a cage at the zoo. I feel like a siren, captivating the women (specifically women) who watch me, and I leave them all begging for my attention.

My fantasy then shifts and I am no longer in the room. I'm in the woods, surrounded by nature. I feel free and liberated, and I feel the energy of the trees and the earth around me. I'm alone, but I don't feel scared – I seem connected to the vitality of the environment, and I feel a deep peace within myself. The sun is setting and I'm standing in a clearing, admiring the beauty of the setting sun. Then I hear a noise coming from the woods. I peer into the darkness and I see a beautiful white horse emerging from the shadows. I gasp in surprise, my heart racing. The horse is stunning, and it seems to be watching me, like it knows me. I am captivated. I take a step closer, and the horse lets me approach. I stroke its mane, and it nuzzles me in response. I feel its energy calming my mind and my body. It arouses me. I climb on the horse's back and it starts to move, taking me on a ride through the woods. I feel like I'm flying as the horse gallops with such grace and strength. I feel my growing erection start to rub on the horse's back and I grow impossibly harder. I feel like staying on this ride forever, and I feel a deep connection with the horse and the surrounding nature. Eventually, we arrive at an isolated lake, and the horse stops and kneels down, giving me a perfect view of the water and the sky. As I watch the sun dip below the horizon, I see a silhouette of a woman emerge from the shadows. She is tall and handsome, and she's wearing a black suit with a red tie. I feel my heart pounding in my chest. I know this woman is here for me.

She walks towards me, and as she gets closer I can see her eyes. They are green, like two deep pools of emeralds. She takes my hands in hers and kisses me on the forehead. Her lips are warm and gentle, and I can't help but relax into her embrace. The woman whispers something in my ear, but I can't seem to hear what she's saying. She whispers again. She's asking me if we could make love. She's asking me for consent. It's something my partner rarely does verbally. Usually, they just start kissing me, and if I shy away, then they stop. But being asked by this woman feels exhilarating. My body responds to her words, and I can feel my desire rising. I want her so badly. The woman leads me away from the lake, and we walk through the woods until we reach an open field. The night sky is filled with stars, and a warm breeze rustles through the grass. She lays me down on the grass and starts to undress me. As she uncovers my body, a wave of warmth spreads through me. She kisses my neck and my shoulders and caresses my body with her thin hands. I'm trembling in anticipation as she moves down to my waist. The woman then kisses my stomach and my inner thighs, and I can feel my body responding to her touch. I want her, and I want her now. She then pulls out a large onion and rubs it across my erection, and the sensation is incredible. I feel an electric current running through me and I'm lost in ecstasy. The woman then moves up my body, and she starts to make love to me. She moves slowly, making sure to pleasure me with every thrust.

I feel more connected to her with each passing moment, and I can feel my body responding to her movements. She is gentle, yet passionate, and I feel like I'm in heaven.

I guess this is what I have always craved in my relationships; the feeling of being small and cherished. Afterwards, as we lie under the stars, I feel completely content and satisfied. I feel like I just experienced something magical and I am truly happy.

As I slowly return to reality, I feel a great sense of peace. In my bed, soaking wet by now, I get the urge to talk to my partner. But I never do. I just lie there, basking in the feeling of being safe and loved.

[Indigenous Moldovan • Orthodox Christian • <$19,000 • Asexual • Cohabiting • Yes]

I read Nancy Friday's *My Secret Garden* in my twenties and again in my forties. Now, in my sixties, it suddenly all makes sense. I'm splayed on a forest floor, hillside or beach. All the animals are watching. Cunnilingus – never coitus – from one/ all/any of the animals. A current favourite seems to be a deer. Sometimes I'm a landscape, with a river gushing through me.

[Mixed Anglo-Indian English • Lapsed Catholic • <$64,000 • Heterosexual • Married/in a civil partnership • Yes]

I wander in an immense forest at night, wearing a simple old-fashioned dress that hangs down to my calves. It's threadbare and vaguely medieval-looking. The ancient trees tower over me, and their long branches rustle in a light wind, as if they're whispering their secrets. The bark is cushioned in thick green moss. I glide my fingers over their tiny phyllids, feel them catching at my skin as if they are trying to lure me closer. Although I am on my own, at night, I am not afraid. Even in the village I wouldn't venture outside my cottage after dark but there is nothing to fear in these woods. Nothing I cannot handle. I enjoy this feeling. The air is thick with the scents of moss, decaying leaves, the rich earthy notes of the dark soil clinging to my bare feet, and something crisp and green. The darkness beneath the trees is sheltered and feels velvety soft against the bare skin of my legs. I hear the beating of hooves and my heart starts to pound. They are coming. Arousal shivers through me and I feel myself growing slick. A group of fauns has found me. They are young men from the knees up, if you ignore the fur on their haunches, but they have hooves instead of feet. Their chests and faces look human, but a set of horns curls up from long, thick hair and their pointed ears are so soft to the touch. Their chests are broad, and they are breathing hard. They must have scented me and come running. 'Don't go into the woods!' girls are cautioned. Every few months, the fauns roam ever closer to the village to try and lure a woman into the darkness, to sport with them. Nobody is taken against their will, but the whole village pretends that the fauns are a danger. 'Stay away! Don't go out at night!' The only monsters, however, are the men prowling the village in a drunken stupor. Some women don't heed the warnings. Nobody mentions the little half-faun babies born every few years. Nothing bad will happen to me. I know the fauns. Ever since I was old enough, I have run into the woods. We meet every few months for a little time away from my drab village life. For a splash of joy in my days. One of them, the one I trust the most, steps into the ring they have formed around me. 'Who do you desire this night?' He is young, about my age, and we met on his first run in the forest – his first and mine. His eyes are chocolate brown, his gaze so warm I want nothing more than to grab his hand and take him home with me. I bite my lip, undecided. Someone new or him? I know it is my choice. And sometimes I have strayed. But today I will pick him. Awareness twinkles in his eyes, even before I say his name. 'I need you,' I whisper, so hungry for him that I reach out and drag him towards me. He is erect, his cock pressing against my soft belly, he lets out a groan of need. I turn round and press into the green cushion of moss. My juices run out of me and down my legs. He leans against my back, rubs his hardness through my slippery centre. But still we wait. Today, he is not enough. There is someone missing. Galloping hooves announce another group of fauns. They carry a woman whom they stole in some other village. Her long brown hair flies behind her like a messy cloud. Her cheeks are rosy from excitement and her eyes glint with arousal. We don't speak, but when they set her down next to me, she takes my hand. She leans back against the tree, facing the fauns, a mirror to my pose, while we each are conquered by a faun. They are big, filling us so well, and I inhale the soft pants of joy that fly from her lips. We both soon moan from the skilful thrusts. My faun growls as he digs his fingers into my hips, anchoring me, keeping me safe. I am me, being fucked so well, cradled in the velvet night of the forest. But I am also the faun ravishing the woman next to me. It is my cock that splits her soft mound. My legs that force her silky thighs further apart. She moans when I thrust into her. Her eyes fly open, staring into mine. They are wide and dreamy with lust. We drink in the sight of each other, while her tight, wet pussy clasps me. Lust sings through our bodies. We have become part of the forest, part of the night, swallowing down the magic all around us. I feel her flutter against my cock and I know she is close. It's like a fever licking me from the base of the skull to my tailbone, a hot flush, knowing that I am making her come, I am making her sigh and dance on my cock. I pull her close for a kiss and we both shatter. I am pulled back into my own body, hear the faun's harsh groan next to my ear, feel him tremble as he spills deep inside me and takes me with him into bliss. We are carried through the dark forest, nuzzled contentedly by the fauns, their strong hearts beating under our cheeks. They drop her off at her village, then blindfold me so I cannot find the way back to her while we are in the harsh light of day. With a sigh and a kiss, they leave me at the edge of the village. 'Don't go,' I whisper, clinging to my faun. He leans his head against mine. 'You are not ready yet.' I will see them again the next time. When I long for the sheltering forest I feel that I am crawling out of my skin with need.

[White German • Lapsed German Protestant • <$64,000 • Bisexual/pansexual • Married/in a civil partnership • Yes]

My deep-seated fantasy, the one to which I touch myself after a warm cup of camomile and milk to bless my dreams, is for a man to be indelibly – and entirely ordinarily – nice to me. I do not long for flowers and speeches and thoughtful presents, nor a vacation at great expense. In my fantasy, I am not spoiled. The thought to which I grow wettest is of a partner who takes care of me in bed, who aims to make our bodies and their pleasure mutually familiar, who is accomplishing all of that niceness in the most generic sense of that term. A friend once spoke of affection dosed out like medicine, carefully counted out on another's palm before it's handed over, reluctantly, begrudgingly. I have known that too, and my fantasy is the opposite. I want to wake up next to someone who lets me press my face into the hollow of his neck. I want him to tell me I feel soft in the morning while he slowly trails his warm touch down my body. He'll take his time reaching my clit, gentle as he waits for me to grow wet for him. Then he'll pull back, look me in the eye as he licks my juices off each of his spread fingers. I want him to move inside me slowly, pausing at intervals to trail his fingers down the inside of my arms. I have known partners who leave me to come down from sex alone; one who pulled up his trousers as soon as his forty-minute timer went off.

In my fantasy, I lead my sex partner to the bath, where I wash my crusted come off his beard, and he cleans his mess from my stomach, the leftovers I have not managed to greedily scoop into my mouth with my fingers. We kiss until we're sudsy and clean. In my fantasy, I want to visit the market together. He'll enquire what I ate yesterday, an uninteresting and mundane detail you have to care about me deeply to want to elicit. Only my mother has ever asked me that. He'll feed me chunks of Honeycrisp apples they've put out as samples, whispering to me that I taste sweeter. At the bookstore nearby, I will tell him about the texts I'm working through simultaneously but slowly, and he'll ask my thoughts on the American South and whether plot is dead in favour of character-building. He'll purchase a book to read because I said it transformed my ethical thinking when I was sixteen, and following our discussion, he'll dig in his phone to send me articles he thinks I might enjoy. He'll say he loves my mind. At home, I will burn the eggs and chard from the market because he's pressed me against the counter. This time will be more urgent. He'll throw the windows open and say he doesn't care who hears. (One previous partner always covered my mouth with his hand.) My fantasy partner will sit on top of me and ask me to tell him exactly what I want. He'll tease my nipples and my clit gently, refusing to touch me firmly until I've laid it all out. I'll be frantic at this point, but he'll ask exactly where to bite, whether I want him to kiss up the inside of my thighs after he satisfies my request to slap them. He'll give me everything I say, pressing one hand down from outside at the spot just above my pelvic bone that makes me scream when paired with his rhythmic, curled fingers inside me. He'll ask if I'm OK; if this is what I imagined. I'll finish by squirting all over his arm. I'll be so loud that I can no longer look my neighbours in the eye. He won't hurry away. He won't hurry at all.

[Asian Chinese • Heterosexual • Single • No]

My fantasy is to have a man love me for who I am and not to see me as a living sex toy.

[African American • >$128,000 • Heterosexual • Single • No]

My biggest fantasy is something not quite typical, especially not alongside the saucy somethings others will be dishing out. Well, my fantasy is for something meaningful. Don't get me wrong, all sex is amazing – believe me, I've been there! But one thing I have missed in my sex life is genuine affection: not just a brush-off and goodbye after he's finished and you're left unsatisfied yet again. Something warm, something you'd find with someone who cares about you. That's all I want.

[Mixed-race British • Atheist • <$19,000 • Bisexual/pansexual • Single • No]

My greatest fantasy is a bit of a fairy tale. I think of myself walking in a tropical rainforest. After a while I find myself in an open space with a lake and a waterfall. Feeling unseen and free, I take off my clothes and dive into the clear water. I get out and lie in the sun to dry. Listening to the sounds of the forest, slowly I fall asleep. I wake up to the touch of several hands and kisses on my skin. I open my eyes and see a couple of naked women adoring my body and pleasuring each other. I lie perfectly still and close my eyes again and let myself go, revelling in a great feeling of happiness and sensuality. I'm getting increasingly turned on when I feel one of the women parting my legs, then start languorously to lick and kiss my pussy. It feels so good that I quickly lose my sense of time and place. When I'm about to come, I open my eyes again to watch her going down on me, and when I see her looking back at me with big green eyes, she makes me orgasm in an explosion of lust and bliss. Waves of desire rush through my body, making my pussy come over and over again. It feels like nothing I ever felt before ...

[Dutch • Atheist • Bisexual/pansexual • Married/in a civil partnership • Yes]

In my fantasy, she takes me to a beautiful garden on an island where there is no one other than us, and we make love vulnerably. She attaches her transforming alien genitalia to my privates; hers take the shape of a sucking lotus flower that stimulates my private parts, then a shiny holographic shaft with which she penetrates me until we both reach our climax. Afterwards we lie there on our picnic blanket in the sun slightly obscured by the beautiful trees in the garden, just looking at each other, with so much love. Her skin is glowing from the sweat of the lovemaking and her eyes and naked body look so hypnotising and beautiful. We make love like this every time we feel like it and just enjoy life.

[Guatemalan Finnish • Pagan • <$19,000 • Homo-romantic Bisexual/pansexual • Single • No]

In a garden, I am perched on a smooth brick pillar. He placed me there, lifted me up. My shirt is open, breasts exposed. I slowly take one breast and clench it tight, feeling my nipple harden as thoughts of tongues and legs spread flood my mind. My back arched, his fingers slip inside of me, so easily. Heavy breath moist in the cold air. I cradle his head as his noises join the symphony of bird life, innocently perched and watching. He opens me, wanting to get deeper, tongue in a pressure-dance as I let out a moan and thrust forward, his hair clenched in needy fists. My fingers move inside and then easily slip across the small, soon to be throbbing mound. Faster. Harder. Waterfalls cascade. I breathe out.

[White Australian • <$64,000 • Heterosexual • In a relationship • Yes]

My absolute favourite fantasy is unfortunately never ever going to happen as it involves a room that I access through my full-length mirror where I am waiting for myself. No, I am not a narcissist (although a narcissist may well say that) – I just love the idea of being totally free to experiment with someone who knows me as well as I know myself, needing no mood-interfering guidance and feeling that total lack of self-consciousness. In my most visited fantasy scenario, I am standing naked in front of my mirror looking at the woman beckoning me with a look of lust and desire like I'm the hottest, baddest bitch in the world. We slowly look over each other's bodies in anticipation. I imagine touching her. I want to make her feel good and she me. I step through the mirror into my naked self's arms; we kiss long and slow, pressing our bodies together, feeling the softness of our breasts against each other. We gently touch each other, with no rush to get off, just enjoying the sensations. Softly kissing, blowing and licking up and down each other's backs and necks, the backs of the thighs, inner thighs, stomachs, without being self-conscious about any wobbles or stretch marks, knowing exactly what the other likes, how to tease – we are identical and understand each other perfectly. Hands and mouths moving soft and slow, brushing against nipples and labia. Breathing getting heavy, getting wet and swollen as we gently suck and bite the nipples, rub the clitoris, tease the vagina by entering only a little, flicking the fingers around the entrance, building to slow, full penetration: in and out, fingers wriggling, tongue flicking the clit. No rush; taking time; knowing when to hold back until we can resist no more and joining clit to clit, sliding over each over, sucking nipples until we climax together but do not stop. Increasing the pressure, moving faster until we climax again, then we lie stroking each other's sensitive stomachs, backs, necks, thighs, before I return back through the mirror to my own world.

[White British • Atheist • <$38,000 • Bisexual or pansexual • Married/in a civil partnership • Yes]

I am thirty-eight years old. For the first time two weeks ago, I had an out-of-body meditative experience where I was making out with myself. I had a vision of myself on top of myself, kissing myself and loving myself for my existence. I got to the point of orgasm while turning myself on, embracing and loving all of me. Seeing all the parts of me that other people see when they are with me intimately. It was a transient and breathtakingly beautiful experience. At nearly forty years of age, I am finally learning to love and accept *all* of me – from the small inner parts to the big luscious outer parts. I am loving the inner child who was hurt, who felt misunderstood, who was taken advantage of and felt frozen in a world of sex and guys, and sex as a whole. Now, I am proud to be a woman who adores sex in all its glory – the energy, the magnitude, the filth, the raunch, the tenderness, the joy, the licking, the holding, the rawness of bodies, the stillness and calmness of spirits and minds, and every fucking ruthless and enthralling moment.

From a young age, I knew sex held a magnificent joy to it. Stealing *The Joy of Sex* from my best friend's parents, the two of us read it in the bushes behind her house, we researched the shit out of that book. Then I asked a crush two years my senior to take me home for lunch so I could practise improving my hand- and blowjobs on him. I had a desire to be good at desiring. But now I am on my self-love journey and I want love in all its raw and real forms. I think of a lover who fucks me from behind, tenderly and passionately. A lustful threesome. Two women, one man. Two men, one woman. I want someone to tie me up in a dungeon and whip my ass; I want someone to do nude yoga with me; I want to do a nude photo shoot; I want to practise tantric sex.

Now that I have finally taken back my body and will no longer let the assault of my past take that place of pleasure from my future, I want to verbalise my sexual desires so I hear them, so the universe hears them, and so others hear them and respect them and perhaps we will all start to speak safely and honestly and truthfully; so that we learn of the beauty, realness and normality of ours sexual desires and pleasures. She desires to roar, and gasp and groan and sigh, and to release and vibrate … and she will have those moments; because she is *I*, and I am the keeper of her.

[White Canadian • Spiritual • <$38,000 • Heterosexual • Single • No]

Here is just an aside. Just its arm around my shoulder and its eyes telling me 'I am here.' I finally allow myself to let go. Just a distance that finally cancels, our two bodies finally touching. Just a hug in which I lose myself. I breathe deeply and close my eyes. Just a reassuring, comforting embrace. I nestle my face in its neck, my lips rest on its skin. I feel its heart beating fast. I stand still, torn between the desire to go further and the fear that reason will prevail. The noises of the street call me back to reality, but I don't want to go back. I stay there, motionless, savouring the seconds that tick away. Just its breathing changing and me straightening up. Just my hands hanging on its waist. Just its hands caressing my forehead. Its fingers slide between my hair, behind my ears, to my neck. Its eyes plunged in mine and a smile. No words, just softness, caresses. Just a kiss on my forehead, my cheek. Just its gaze trying to decipher me and my smile telling it 'Yes, you can continue.' Just its lips approaching, hesitating, and brushing my mouth. Just its lips on mine and the heat. Just our tongues touching and gently uncovering each other. In the depths of my being, butterflies come to life. Its arms embrace me, squeeze me. I feel so good. Just its hands passing under my shirt. Its fingers sliding down my spine. With calm and respect. Just its steps leading me to the sofa, its kisses intensifying. Just its body on mine, our limbs adjusting. Just its dark eyes probing me. I take off my top, and its one, too. I want to feel its skin against mine. Just its lips running down my neck, my chest. Its smell takes me away. Let time stand still. *Carpe diem.* My worries disappear, my responsibilities as a mother, a wife, a worker disappear: just me and what is deepest in me. Just shoes coming off and two pairs of trousers falling to the floor. Just its mouth on my breasts and the desire rising in me. The happiness, the well-being intoxicates me. Its long hair brushes my stomach. Its nose caresses me below the navel. I have shivers but I am not cold. Its kisses are little bits of heaven. Just underwear ripping off. Its head comes down between my thighs. I grab its hands and squeeze them hard. I'm hot, I want to cry, I can hardly breathe. Just its tongue exploring me and my heart exploding. I fly away, I leave, I leave everything, I forget everything. I am flying, time has stopped. Just a bit of madness in my well-ordered life. Just Her and me. She is my folly, my time for me. She is my unconfessed desire, my repressed thoughts. She is my forbidden, my secret. She is a gift, an indelible trace. She is an unhoped-for moment. She is part of my path, of my history. She does not share my daily life, my home, but she is my parenthesis. She is just her.

[White French • Atheist • <$64,000 • Heterosexual • Married/in a civil partnership • Yes]

Lying on a sandy shore, the waves stroke me slowly as they break over my thighs and hips. When they retreat, they leave flowers blooming on my skin.

[White British • Atheist • <$38,000 • Bisexual/pansexual • In a relationship • No]

a note on Gillian Anderson

Gillian Anderson is an award-winning film, television and theatre actor, producer and director. Among other honours, she has won two Primetime Emmy Awards, two Golden Globe Awards, three Screen Actors Guild Awards and an *Evening Standard* Theatre Award. In addition to her acting work, Gillian is also globally recognised as a respected activist and charity campaigner, previously co-authored the *Sunday Times* bestseller *We: A Manifesto for Women Everywhere* with Jennifer Nadel, and in 2023 founded the wellness drinks brand G-Spot which encourages women to embrace their unique power. In 2016 Anderson was appointed an honorary OBE (Order of the British Empire) for her services to drama. She lives in London with her three children.